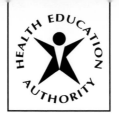

Effectiveness of interventions to promote healthy eating in pregnant women and women of childbearing age: a review

Edwin R van Teijlingen
Brenda J Wilson
Nessa Barry
Ann Ralph
Geraldine McNeill
Wendy Graham
Doris Campbell

Series Editor Jane Meyrick

HEA Project Team

Jane Meyrick   Research Project Manager
Antony Morgan   Head of Monitoring and Effectiveness Research

In the same series:

Health promotion in older people for the prevention of coronary heart disease and stroke

Health promotion in childhood and young adolescence for the prevention of unintentional injuries

Effectiveness of video for health education

Effectiveness of mental health promotion interventions

Health promotion with young people for the prevention of substance misuse

Health promotion interventions to promote healthy eating in the general population

Effectiveness of oral health promotion

Effectiveness of interventions to promote healthy feeding of infants under one year: a review

Effectiveness of interventions to promote healthy eating in preschool children aged 1–5 years: a review

Effectiveness of interventions to promote healthy eating in elderly people living in the community: a review

Effectiveness of interventions to promote healthier living in people from minority ethnic groups: a review

Forthcoming topics:

Health promotion interventions in the workplace: a review

Opportunities for and barriers to change in dietary behaviour in elderly people

Opportunities for and barriers to change in dietary behaviour in minority ethnic groups

Opportunities for and barriers to good nutritional health in women of childbearing age, pregnant women, infants under 1 and children aged 1 to 5

© Health Education Authority, 1998

ISBN 0 7521 1097 7

Health Education Authority
Trevelyan House
30 Great Peter Street
London SW1P 2HW

Designed by Edwin Belchamber
Typeset by Wayzgoose
Cover design by Maria Grasso
Printed in Great Britain

Effectiveness of interventions to promote healthy eating in pregnant women and women of childbearing age: a review

Contents

Acknowledgements

Acknowledgements are due to the following people who contributed to this project by providing information, support, expertise or encouragement: Helen Adamson, Angela Bradley, Julie Bruce, Lynn Conway, Catriona Crosswaite, Lorna Cummings, Margaret Didcock, Charlotte Evans, Margaret Forest, Adrian Grant, Jeremy Grimshaw, Emma Harvey, Fiona Hogarth, Morag Macritchie, Moira Napper, Dean Phillips, Wendy Pirie, Margaret Reid, Ian Ronald, Elizabeth Russell, Paul Sparks, Cathy Steer, Rosel Talloch, Sheila Wallace, Stuart Watson, Emma Witney and Wendy Wrieden.

Structure of the report

The report begins with a short introductory preface by the HEA to put the report into context of its position in the series.

The report is then divided into three main sections: an executive summary, the main report, and appendices.

The *executive summary* briefly outlines the objectives and methods of the review, followed by the main findings and conclusions.

The *main report* begins by providing a background to the promotion of healthy eating for women and women of childbearing age, the aims and objectives are identified in greater detail and methodology and scope of the review outlined. The report then presents the results of the review with detailed information about all the studies included and discusses innovative studies excluded on the grounds of methodological rigour. This is followed by the detailed discussion and conclusions of the findings on effectiveness.

The *technical appendices* provide details of the full methodology, including data extraction forms and search strategy as well as full summary tables of characteristics and findings of each study. This is followed by a commentary on the North American WIC Program, and a list of studies located, but not included, in the review.

Preface

The Health Education Authority (HEA) welcomes this new review of effectiveness of healthy eating interventions to promote healthy eating in pregnant women and women of childbearing age as one means of gathering evidence for health promotion. It forms one of an HEA series of systematic reviews that have begun to address the need for an evidence base in health promotion. This report provides an exhaustive review of the available evidence and highlights the importance for health promoters not only to evaluate their work but to evaluate it well, in order to increase the body of work reviews can draw on.

This report is one in a set of linked reviews within the HEA series of effectiveness reviews of health promotion interventions which examine healthy eating in various populations. The need to focus on these populations was identified in an earlier review in the HEA series examining healthy eating in the general population[1] but is also in response to the findings of previous reviews that health promotion work is more effective if targeted at specific population groups.

This report is published alongside a set of sister reviews, of 'Opportunities for and barriers to change' in the same target groups, commissioned by the Department of Health[2] to examine the behavioural patterns, attitudes and cultural values which might provide opportunities for, or constitute barriers to, healthy eating. The two sets of reviews are complementary in their scope and coverage of the literature and while individual studies may appear in more than one review, they are covered from different perspectives.

The aim of systematic reviews

The commitment within the NHS to move towards evidence-based practice has, to some extent, been mirrored within health promotion. For this reason the methodological tool used to find evidence, the systematic review, has been applied to a range of health promotion topics in an effort to inform health professionals in addition to increasing the knowledge base about effective health promotion.

[1]Roe *et al.* (1997). *Health promotion interventions to promote healthy eating in the general population: a review*. London: Health Education Authority.

[2]Reid *et al.* (1998). *Opportunities for and barriers to good nutritional health in women of childbearing age, pregnant women, infants under 1 and children aged 1 to 5*. London: Health Education Authority.

Executive summary

A systematic review of the published English language literature was conducted in order to answer the following research questions:

(a) do women of childbearing age and women who are pregnant change their dietary knowledge, attitudes and/or behaviour in response to specific interventions?

(b) what is the extent of such changes (if any)?

(c) what are the characteristics of interventions (if any) which appear to be effective?

The review followed the methodology of the Cochrane Collaboration and the NHS Centre for Reviews and Dissemination; it focused on identifying and assessing rigorous evaluations of interventions designed to promote a healthier diet in participants as described above. A sensitive search strategy was developed and applied to a number of electronic databases including MEDLINE, EMBASE and health education/health promotion and social science databases; relevant articles were also identified by hand-searching key journals, checking reference lists of reports and consulting with relevant researchers and specialists. Reports identified in this way were each scrutinised by two independent reviewers and included or excluded according to defined criteria; structured information on study design, type of participants and type of intervention was extracted from each report which fulfilled the inclusion criteria. Data on outcomes from each report were collated and analysed to produce a comprehensive overview of the changes in specific dietary indicators achieved as a result of the interventions.

Summary of main findings

The search strategy identified a total of 585 reports covering the two target groups; of these, 71 were formally assessed and the remainder were excluded on the basis of the abstract. A total of ten reports, giving details of nine studies, fulfilled the inclusion criteria and contributed to the formal analysis (five studies in women of childbearing age and four in women who were pregnant). Of these, seven were randomised controlled trials, one was a non-randomised, controlled before-and-after study and in one it was unclear whether the control group was allocated randomly or not. Many of the studies were subject to bias, particularly lack of observer blinding, and using assessment tools of unknown validity.

All five interventions assessed in women of childbearing age were community-based; two appeared to be predominantly educational (one involving a video supplemented by printed material, the other involving a series of nutrition lessons), two involved an exercise programme (one strength training alone, the other as part of a wider intervention also involving education and peer support) and one was described as offering empowerment and support to new mothers. The duration of these interventions varied from a single session to regular meetings for at least a year.

Taken together, these studies suggest that participants can improve their knowledge and dietary intake, particularly fat intake, and that the changes are statistically significantly greater in groups receiving an intervention compared with the controls. Insufficient data were obtained to comment on whether the changes are sustained. This, along with the diversity of the interventions and methodological flaws in some of the evaluations make it difficult to identify interventions which are likely to be successful if more widely applied.

Of the four interventions in pregnant women, two were community-based and two were clinic-based. All had an educational component and in three this was enhanced by counselling and/or psychosocial support of varying degrees. One of the interventions involved distributing printed material at the clinic booking appointment and mailing a second pack at 26 weeks' gestation; the others consisted of a number of contacts throughout the second half of pregnancy.

Only one study in pregnant women provided specific outcome data in relation to a healthy diet as defined in this review; it had adequate statistical power and demonstrated small improvements in both control and intervention groups, with a greater, but statistically non-significant, improvement in the intervention group. This study also evaluated changes in knowledge and attitudes and demonstrated small changes in the desired direction in control and intervention groups; the difference in knowledge scores between the groups reached statistical significance but the magnitude of the difference is unlikely to represent an improvement which is worthwhile in practice. The other three studies suggested that pregnant women appear to improve their intake of energy and possibly protein in response to interventions designed to improve pregnancy outcomes, but they did not provide data on other components of a healthy diet or on knowledge or attitudes. Taken together, it is not possible to conclude whether or not healthy eating interventions in pregnancy are effective.

Conclusions

We conclude that women of childbearing age, and women who are pregnant, may be responsive to interventions designed to promote healthy eating. However, the evidence is insufficiently robust to recommend immediate implementation of the interventions without further, more rigorous, evaluations to assess the repeatability of the findings, the true magnitude of the changes and whether they are sustained over time.

The rationale for healthy eating interventions in pregnancy needs to be clarified, particularly whether there is good epidemiological evidence that increasing the intake of particular nutrients and energy is of benefit in healthy women and their infants.

1. Introduction

Background

This report was commissioned by the Health Education Authority as part of a set of related systematic reviews of interventions to promote healthy eating in particular population groups. This review concentrated on interventions aimed at women of childbearing age and women who are pregnant.

The importance of promoting healthy eating in pregnant women and women of childbearing age

There are many reasons for promoting healthy eating in women. Despite living longer, women have worse health than men (World Health Organization, 1992), and nutrition is believed to play a part in many of the leading causes of illness and death in women – for example, coronary heart disease and stroke, breast and large bowel cancers, osteoporosis and diabetes. Looking across the reproductive lifecycle, healthy diet has been linked with onset of menarche and bone development in adolescent girls; in non-pregnant women, menstrual dysfunctions such as amenorrhea and premenstrual syndrome have been studied in relation to numerous nutritional factors, including body weight, low-fat, high complex carbohydrate diets, and micro-nutrient imbalance (Doyle, 1996). It is, however, the relationship between women's reproductive role and nutrition which has been the subject of more extensive research over many years. Within this, the focus of attention has usually been on achieving positive health outcomes in the foetus or infant rather than the woman herself, and on nutritional supplementation rather than healthy eating per se. As we discuss below, however, the benefits of improving the dietary habits of women who are pregnant or of childbearing age reach beyond the improved maternal, foetal and infant health, to the health of other family members (children and adults) and future generations.

Maternal nutrition is important for the foetus
Adequate nutrition in a pregnant woman is important to allow her foetus to grow and develop physically and mentally to its full potential. At each stage in development, all nutrients are required at ideal levels. Adequate protein is essential but high protein diets have disadvantages (Kramer,

1993). It is now well recognised that, in the early weeks, folate is crucial to neural tube development (MRC, 1991) but it has also been suggested that deficiency of folate at later stages may result in abortion or low birthweight (Baumslag et al., 1970). Iron is important to prevent anaemia and for normal brain development; normal intelligence also depends on adequate iodine. Vitamin A is important for the development of the eye and for general growth. Vitamin D is required to prevent osteomalacia, and long chain fatty acids from fish oils are important in brain development and in increasing the length of gestation so allowing a greater birthweight (Olsen et al., 1992). A baby born at full term weighing over 2.5 kg is likely to suffer less illness and grow more steadily than a baby of lower birthweight, who is more vulnerable to infections and may have difficulty feeding (Ruys-Dudok et al., 1989; Skeoch et al., 1989; Ens-Dokkum et al., 1992).

Foetal growth and birthweight may influence adult health

Recent evidence (Barker, 1992, 1994) also suggests that not only birthweight but also disproportionate foetal growth (for example the larger placenta that develops as a response to anaemia (Godfrey et al., 1995)) may have long-term effects. Smaller babies are more at risk of heart disease in later life and the disproportionate placenta predisposes to hypertension (Edwards et al., 1993). Diabetes and obesity have both been related to inappropriate foetal growth. There is also evidence of intergenerational effects of foetal gonadal developments. Animal studies suggest that the ovum may be programmed by the mother's nutritional state, even before implantation (Wallace, Aitken and Cheyne, 1994).

Mothers have their own nutritional needs

Good nutrition is also important to the mother herself, at a time when she is vulnerable. She needs to have sufficient energy and appropriate levels of nutrients to maintain her own health as well as provide for the foetus and her future breastfeeding needs (Rush, 1986). A pregnant woman needs to keep fit and active, avoid hazards from food (for example infections and specific hypervitaminoses), maintain a healthy immune system, maintain her blood pressure and avoid anaemia. A teenager who is pregnant is at special risk: she may not have completed her own growth, so her physical needs may compete with those of the foetus, to the detriment of both (Fraser, Brockert and Wand, 1995).

Women of childbearing age may be several weeks' pregnant before they realise their condition and before they can make a conscious decision to improve their diet for the sake of their baby. The early stages of pregnancy are critical and nutrient deficiencies in the first few weeks can have permanent and irreversible effects (for example folate deficiency causing neural tube defects). It is therefore important that women eat a healthy diet before pregnancy. The weight of the mother before pregnancy, as well as her weight gain during pregnancy, can affect the birthweight of the baby (World Health Organization, 1995). In women seeking to become pregnant, healthy eating is argued to affect not only conception and early spontaneous abortion, but also the outcome at term (Bendich and Keen, 1993).

Women of childbearing age often feed the family

Apart from the importance of diet in the health of mother and foetus, it should also be remembered that women of childbearing age occupy a central position in making dietary decisions for whole families. The woman not only feeds herself and her baby, she also makes decisions for older children in the family and (often) her partner or other adults in the household. Research has shown that mothers are key to the establishment of healthy eating patterns of their children, that calcium intake by children mirrors that of their mothers, and when women adopt diets lower in fat content, partners often follow suit. Eating patterns adopted by a mother of young children may have an effect on the whole family and set patterns for future generations.

Given these arguments, it is argued that nutrition counselling of women of reproductive age can have far-reaching implications (Bowman and Spangler, 1995). Pregnancy is seen as a particularly suitable time for encouraging dietary change as women often modify their diets at this time owing to physical symptoms; they may be more responsive to health advice, they often actively seek health information and the antenatal care system provides an opportunity to reach large numbers of women (Anderson, 1996). In addition to advice specific to pregnancy, arguments have been made to include counselling to reduce dietary cholesterol (NCEP, 1993), to maintain an adequate lifetime calcium intake (NIH, 1994), and to encourage higher daily fruit and vegetable intakes to protect against a number of cancers (Block, 1992).

Women themselves recognise the importance of healthy eating – for example, when a sample of women were asked the question, 'What is the most important thing people can do to promote long-term good health?', the most popular response was 'Eating a healthy diet' (Flynn, 1996). This perception is built up from a range of sources – from women's magazines to dietary guidelines, and from lay persons to health professionals. However, as with many health promotion activities, questions remain as to the effectiveness of interventions which are targeted at behaviour change. It is the purpose of this review to describe the range of interventions evaluated in recent years and to assess the available well-founded research evidence on whether they are effective, in order to make recommendations for policy and for future research in this area.

2. Aims and objectives

Aims

Based on a comprehensive synthesis of the current published English language evidence, the aims of this review are to determine:

- whether women of childbearing age and women who are pregnant change their dietary knowledge, attitudes and/or behaviour in response to specific interventions

- the extent of such changes (if any)

- the characteristics of the interventions (if any) which appear to be effective.

The objectives

The objectives are to identify:

- the extent of the reported change in intake of key dietary indicators in participants (experimental and control) in studies fulfilling the inclusion criteria

- quantitative differences in the size of changes in intake of key dietary indicators in the two types of participants (women of childbearing age and women who are pregnant)

- the characteristics of effective interventions, as far as reported details allow

- specific issues in the design and evaluation of future interventions aimed at improving knowledge, attitudes and behaviour in these target groups

- specific research questions which remain to be addressed.

3. Methods

Methodology

We took the approach of a systematic review, with relevant studies identified by systematic searching and independently assessed for relevance to the review. Data on study design and results were systematically extracted from studies fulfilling inclusion criteria. The heterogeneity of interventions, target groups, study designs and statistical techniques meant that full meta-analysis of the results was impossible. Instead, we have provided a narrative review and presented summary information in tables. Studies reporting interventions which were evaluated in an insufficiently rigorous manner are listed for completeness but were not fully reviewed or tabulated. Full details of the methodology are given in Appendix A.

Definitions used in the review

We adopted the following definition of *health promotion*: 'any planned measure which promotes health or prevents disease, disability and premature death' (Whitehead, 1991). This encompasses health education, counselling, changes in environment and changes in policy. All interventions aimed at improving diet were included, irrespective of whether or not this was the investigators' explicit or implicit primary goal.

We included studies which targeted free-living women of childbearing age and/or pregnant women. By *free-living* we mean not living permanently in institutions, for example prison or hospital. Specifically excluded were studies targeting women at clinically-defined high risk of diet-related disease, for example diabetic women, or malnourished women. We examined interventions for the two target groups separately.

We included studies with the following groups of participants as studies targeting *women of childbearing age*:

- women recruited explicitly because they are of 'childbearing age'
- women of childbearing age (15–45 or thereabouts if not otherwise specified) recruited for other or unspecified reasons
- women of childbearing age/aged 15–45 recruited as part of a study of a wider population of adult women only (i.e. with a proportion of

participants older than childbearing age, but not including males). Where possible, results specific to the subgroup of women with childbearing age were sought.

We defined as *healthy eating* any target outcome broadly in line with the National Advisory Committee on Nutrition Education's (NACNE) 1983 recommendations (NACNE, 1983):

(a) total fat intake of 115 g or less per day (34% of total energy) (i.e. reduction)
(b) an average intake of saturated fatty acids of 50 g or less per day (15% of total energy) (i.e. reduction)
(c) an average intake of polyunsaturated fatty acids of 18 g or more per day (5% of total energy) (i.e. increase)
(d) an intake of less than 30 g of sucrose per day (12% of total energy) (i.e. reduction in sugar intake) (i.e. reduction)
(e) maintenance of energy intake through low-fat foods, particularly bread, potatoes, fruit and vegetables (i.e. increase)
(f) an intake of 25 g or more of dietary fibre per day (i.e. increase)
(g) an intake of 1 g or less of salt per day (i.e. reduction).

Scope

We tried to address the broad question 'how effective are health promotion interventions in promoting healthier eating in women who are pregnant and women of childbearing age?' In practice, the interventions are examined in two settings: health care based, for example clinics, and in the community, for example home environment or a community setting. We restricted the review to studies based on experimental or quasi-experimental designs. By 'effectiveness' we meant a useful change in a health outcome when an intervention is implemented in situations resembling real life, where compliance, for example, may be more difficult to ensure. We therefore concentrated on evaluations conducted in field settings where it is likely that external validity (generalisability) is maximised.

We excluded studies where the aim of the intervention was weight management in overweight subjects, and not at healthy eating per se and studies reporting *the effect of* supplementation with vitamins and other nutrients, which we chose to regard as therapeutic interventions rather than healthy eating. However, our criteria did not exclude reports of interventions designed to *prevent obesity* in non-obese subjects, or reports of interventions *to encourage women to consume* appropriate recommended supplementation, for example folic acid supplements in the peri-conceptional period.

We have reviewed separately reports of evaluations of the US Special Supplemental Food Program for Women, Infants and Children (the WIC Program), (Rush *et al.*, 1988 a–e). Very few of these reports fulfilled our methodological inclusion criteria and most of them focused on pregnancy outcomes (for example birthweight) rather than nutrition outcomes. However, we felt that a commentary would be useful both for completeness, and because of the importance and cost of this initiative. This is reported in Appendix E.

4. Results

Search strategy and results of systematic search

The final search strategy is included in Appendix E. The results of the search are summarised in Table 1. A total of 585 published articles were identified including reviews, commentaries and reports of non-intervention studies as well as intervention studies. A large proportion of articles was rejected at the abstract phase as clearly not fulfilling the inclusion criteria. Of the articles which were formally reviewed, around 15 per cent were eventually included.

Table 1: Overall summary of the reports identified

Stage	Results
Primary search	585
First-phase exclusion	514
Wrong target population	411
Wrong intervention or target outcome	97
Unable to obtain a copy	6
Obtained for formal review	71
Second-phase exclusion	49
Not an intervention study	20
Intervention study failed scope criteria	13
Intervention study failed methodological criteria or was duplicate report	16
Included in main review	10
Pregnant women	5*
Women of childbearing age	5
Included in WIC commentary	12

*Includes one intervention study reported in two parts in two articles

Characteristics of studies identified for review

Nine studies (reported in 10 articles) fulfilled the inclusion criteria. The key features of the study designs are detailed in Appendix F and details of the selected dietary measurements are presented in Appendix G. Table 2 shows that most of the studies included in the review are randomised controlled trials (7) with one using a non-randomised control group design and one unclear. No interrupted time series studies were identified. Using sample size as a rough guide to likely power, all studies had an average of at least 20 participants per group and some were much larger. Similarly, using concealment of allocation as an indicator of adequate control of bias, the majority of studies failed to report allocation methods in sufficient detail to allow assessment. The published reports which were obtained for assessment but which did not fulfil inclusion criteria are listed in Appendix H and a short description of the features of some of the interventions is included in this chapter, although no conclusions regarding their effectiveness is possible. The main findings of this report are based on the studies fulfilling the inclusion criteria, which are summarised below. We describe and comment on the nature of the interventions and the evidence of their effectiveness.

Table 2: Characteristics of evaluations fulfilling inclusion criteria

		Women of childbearing age	Women who are pregnant
Evaluation design	Randomised controlled trial	3	4
	Controlled before and after study	1	0
	Unclear whether or not controls randomised	1	0
Sample size in each group	< 20	0	0
	20–49	2	1
	≥ 50	3	3
Concealment of allocation	Adequate	0	2
	Unclear	4	1
	Inadequate	0	1
	Not used	1	0

Details of reports

The key points of each study fulfilling inclusion criteria are described in detail below. Table 3 provides an overview of the characteristics of the interventions evaluated in these studies. No one single approach predominated, but most interventions were education- or counselling-based, most were set in the community and the duration of the intervention ranged from a single one-off session to 6 months or more.

Table 3: Summary of intervention characteristics of included evaluations

		Women of childbearing age	Women who are pregnant
Type	Mainly education	2	1
	Mainly counselling	0	0
	Mixed/enhanced	1	3
	Other	2	0
Setting	Community	5	2
	Clinical	0	2
Duration	Single session	1	0
	Under 12 weeks	0	0
	12 weeks to under 6 months	2	4
	6 to under 12 months	2	0
	12 months and over	0	0

Women of childbearing age – details of interventions and evaluations

Five studies were included which fulfilled the inclusion criteria for this participant group (Table 4). The reported interventions were diverse, with a variety of stated aims – to reduce the risk of specific diseases (cancer (Cox *et al.*, 1995), cardiovascular disease (Brown, Lee and Oyomopito, 1996)), and to improve child health (Johnson, Howell and Molloy, 1993)), as well as to promote a healthier diet as an aim in itself (Fine *et al.*, 1994) or to investigate the dietary behavioural correlates of strength training (Tucker, Harris and Martin, 1996). The studies by Johnson, Howell and Molloy, Fine *et al.* and Cox *et al.* were specifically targeted at women of childbearing age, although not necessarily for reasons of enhancing reproductive health; the studies by Brown, Lee and Oyomopito and Tucker, Harris and Martin were aimed at the general adult female population and included some post-menopausal participants.

Table 4: Summary of rigorously evaluated interventions targeted at women of childbearing age

Study (in order of publication)	Type of intervention	How the intervention was delivered
Johnson, Howell and Molloy (1993)	Empowerment and support	Regular visits by trained volunteer mothers to first-time mothers
Fine *et al.* (1994)	Pre-defined education	One-off educational video showing plus various forms of printed material
Cox *et al.* (1995)	Pre-defined education	Series of community-based nutrition lessons delivered by 'indigenous paraprofessionals'
Brown, Lee and Oyomopito (1996)	Pre-defined education, exercise	Health and fitness group meetings plus home exercise programme and written material
Tucker, Harris and Martin (1996)	Pre-defined exercise programme	Gym-based strength training exercises

Details of individual reports

Johnson, Z, Howell, F and Molloy, B.
Community mothers' programme: randomised controlled trial of non-professional intervention in parenting.
British Medical Journal 1993; **306**:1449–52.

This RCT was carried out in Dublin with participants who were mainly from manual socioeconomic groups. The stated aim of the intervention was to improve development in children born to first-time mothers and consisted of monthly visits by a 'volunteer mother' from the same community who advised and supported her throughout the infant's first year of life. This intervention took place over and above the standard public health nurse support, which formed the control intervention. The basis for the intervention was work carried out by Barker at the University of Bristol Early Childhood Development Unit (Barker, 1984). The authors report that 'the essential feature of this approach is empowerment of the parent', who 'is regarded on equal terms and not given advice by the community mother. Instead the community mother shares her own experiences with the new mother and raises her self-esteem and confidence in herself as a parent'.

The primary outcomes of this study related to child development and nutrition, but maternal nutrition was assessed (using categories of 'appropriate' and 'inappropriate' diet) around the time of the child's first birthday, using the 24-hour recall method.

The study participants were women of childbearing age, who had recently become new mothers. The target outcome was not dietary behaviour in the mother, but in her child, and was part of a wider range of outcomes; by measuring maternal nutrition behaviour, the authors signalled that they considered improvement in the mother's diet a possible by-product of the intervention. This outcome was assessed non-blindly using a standard method and few details are given of the process of categorisation of intakes into 'appropriate' and 'inappropriate' – a crude separation which does not allow for estimation for the extent of the change in intervention mothers. The authors suggest that lack of blinding would be unlikely to lead to observer bias but this should be borne in mind when interpreting any positive findings.

Fine, G A, Conning, D M, Firmin, C, de Looy, A E, Losowsky, M S, Richards, I D G and Webster, J.
Nutrition education of young women.
British Journal of Nutrition 1994; **71**:789–98.

This was a report of a UK-based RCT where the aim of the community-based intervention was the improvement in dietary knowledge in young women in line with COMA recommendations. The participants were young adult women (aged 25–34 years) in socioeconomic groups C2 and D, and the intervention was delivered in the community; no explicit rationale is given for targeting this particular population group. The authors suggest that people need to understood the nutritional basis for healthy eating advice as a prerequisite for behaviour change, and the outcomes of the trial were in terms of nutrition knowledge rather than actual dietary behaviour. Four subgroups of participants were formed according to combinations of assessed 'ability' and 'motivation', prior to the intervention.

Five educational interventions were assessed: a basic nutrition education booklet, a nutrition 'news-sheet', a poster with the same factual content as the booklet (for 'low ability' participants), an educational and 'motivational' video ('test video') featuring a professional entertainer and the same video without the 'motivational' content. It is implied that the educational content was dictated by the recommendations of the NACNE (NACNE, 1983) and similar reports. The primary outcome for the study was improvement in nutrition knowledge one week after the intervention, as assessed by a self-completion instrument.

The experimental group received the test video along with the booklet/poster and news-sheet and a control group received the control video along with the booklet. A further 'baseline' control group did not receive any intervention over and above data collection. The components of the overall package of interventions delivered to the intervention group but not to the control group were therefore the motivation content of the video, the news-sheet and the poster. To assess the effect of the knowledge component of the video and the nutrition booklet it would be necessary to compare the control group with the baseline group.

Regarding the evaluation methodology, a number of points should be noted. Firstly, no indication is given of the smallest change in knowledge that would be considered 'worthwhile' and no sample size calculations are reported. It is therefore unclear whether the differences observed are meaningful, from the authors' perspective. Secondly, it is difficult to disentangle the effects of the different interventions because of the way they were allocated to the test and control groups and the limited reporting of results. Thirdly, it is not clear whether the outcomes data were collected blindly; finally, the inclusion of test group non-attenders in the baseline group for the purposes of analysis introduces bias in favour of the intervention and weakens the pragmatic aspect of the evaluation and the generalisability of the results.

Brown, W J, Lee, C and Oyomopito, R.
Effectiveness of a bilingual heart health program for Greek–Australian women.
Health Promotion International 1996; **11**:117–25.

This reports the findings of a controlled before-and-after study carried out in Australia. The setting was community-based and the participants were adult females aged between 32 and 65 years, of Greek extraction, who were part of a church group. They were of mixed socioeconomic background and not all were bilingual in Greek and English. The primary aim of the intervention was to promote 'heart health' through reducing fat intake and promoting exercise and the programme was specifically designed to be 'minimal intervention' and to overcome language and socio-cultural barriers. The intervention took the form of weekly group meetings for 12 weeks led by health and fitness leaders; these were supplemented by a home-based exercise and dietary programme and printed material. Outcome data were collected from a neighbourhood group which acted as a control.

Outcome data were collected at the end of the intervention with follow-up 12 weeks after that, and took the form of a 'fat habit' questionnaire, anthropometric measurements, serum lipid levels and indicators of fitness. The control data were collected at the beginning and end of a 12-week period.

The study was based on only 48 subjects, so the possibility of inadequate power needs to be considered. Insufficient details are reported to assess the degree of observer bias, although reasonably objective outcome measures were assessed. The choice of a non-randomised control group protected against possible contamination which is important in a community-based project such as this, at the cost of some difference between the groups in baseline socioeconomic indicators; this may have introduced some confounding to the results.

Cox, R H, Parker, G G, Watson, A C, Robinson, S H, Simonson, C J, Elledge, J C, Diggs, S and Smith, M.
Dietary cancer risk of low-income women and change with intervention.
American Dietetic Association Journal 1995; **95**:1031–4.

This reports the results of a trial conducted in the USA, where the explicit aim of the community-based intervention was to improve cancer risk by improving diet. The participants were women aged 20–45 years, on low incomes, some of whom were pregnant. The intervention was part of the US government-funded Virginia Expanded Food and Nutrition Education Program which was already considered effective in improving the diets of low-income families. It consisted of either 10–13 cancer prevention plus nutrition lessons over 6 months, or 9 nutrition-only lessons over 6 months. The control group received 9 money-management lessons over 6 months. The lessons were delivered by 'indigenous paraprofessionals' who taught women in their homes or in small neighbourhood groups. The Health Belief Model provided the theoretical framework for the lessons which incorporated written guidelines, visual aids (flip charts, videos, food models) and hands-on activities. Dietary behaviour outcomes were assessed by 24-hour recall at the end of the intervention period.

The study probably had adequate statistical power but sample size calculations are not reported. It is difficult to judge the methodological quality of the study because details are not reported – in particular it is not clear how participants were allocated to groups and whether outcome data were collected by blinded observers. It is also not clear whether the reported number of participants in each group represents those recruited or those completing the study – as written the results imply zero attrition.

Tucker, L A, Harris, K and Martin, J R.
Participation in a strength training program leads to improved dietary intake in adult women.
American Dietetic Association Journal 1996; **96**:388–90.

This was an RCT based in the USA designed to assess the effect of a strength training programme on energy intake and diet composition (in the absence of a specific dietary intervention). The intervention was set in the community with participants aged between 23 and 66 years, 40 per cent of whom had a college education. It consisted of strength training three times per week for 12 weeks, with a control group receiving flexibility training three times per week for 12 weeks; both groups were advised to consume their usual diet and agreed not to start a weight-reducing diet during the intervention period.

Outcomes were assessed at baseline, 6 and 12 weeks. Changes in diet were assessed by 7-day diaries and anthropometric measurements were made.

While the primary motivation for the trial did not appear to be to assess whether strength training was a useful approach to encouraging improvements in diet (rather it seemed designed to examine the correlation between two physiological variables), the outcomes were directly relevant to this review. The study size was calculated to give adequate power and important details of the methods were reported, suggesting that it was of at least moderate quality. However, there was some potential for positive bias through potentially inadequate blinding and the volunteer nature of the participants limits the generalisability of the findings.

Women of childbearing age – details of outcomes

Table 5 summarises the key outcomes from the five studies included in this category.

One study reported data on knowledge-related outcomes (Fine *et al.*, 1994). All three groups (including the baseline group which received no intervention) showed an improvement in knowledge scores, with a statistically significantly greater improvement in both the test and control groups compared with the baseline group. No difference was observed between the test and control groups. Insufficient details are given to assess whether the within-group before–after changes were each statistically significant or to comment on the likely relative effectiveness of the different components of the interventions.

The authors suggest that further work was planned on whether improvements in knowledge are translated into dietary behaviour changes, but no follow-up publications could be identified at the time of writing.

Table 5: Improvement in key nutrition outcomes in women of childbearing age

Study	Timing of assessment	Extent of change within group following intervention between groups[a]		Absolute difference following intervention
Knowledge				
Fine *et al.* (1994)		Knowledge score	Maximum = 36	
		Control	+2.5[b]	
		Intervention 1	+5.5[b]	+3.4[c]
		Intervention 2	+4.7[b]	+4.5[c]
Attitudes				
No studies reported this outcome				
Behaviour				
Johnson, Howell and Molloy (1993)	1 year = end of intervention	Percentage reporting appropriate intake		
		Wholefoods		
		Control	Not	
		Intervention	estimable	+60[c]
		Vegetables		
		Control	Not	
		Intervention	estimable	+38[c]
		Fruit		
		Control	Not	
		Intervention	estimable	+27[c]
		Energy		
		Control	Not	
		Intervention	estimable	+41[c]
Brown, Lee and Oyomopito (1996)	12 weeks = end of intervention	Fat habit score	Score	
		Control	−0.25	
		Intervention	−0.95[d]	−1.55[c]
		Cholesterol level	mmol/l	
		Control	(+0.11)	
		Intervention	(+0.10)	+0.28
		BMI	kg/m²	
		Control	−0.1	
		Intervention	−1.7[d]	−0.7

[a]Result in brackets indicates direction opposite to desired
[b]Not possible to assess statistical significance of before–after changes
[c]$p < 0.05$ for between-group difference
[d]$p < 0.05$ for change from baseline

Table 5: Improvement in key nutrition outcomes in women of childbearing age (contd)

Study	Timing of assessment	Extent of change within group following intervention between groups[a]		Absolute difference following intervention[a]
Cox et al. (1995)	End of intervention	Daily intake of		
		Energy	kcal	
		Control	(+171)[b]	
		Intervention 1	(+227)[b]	(+56)
		Intervention 2	(+103)[b]	−68
		Fat	% energy	
		Control	−0.3[b]	
		Intervention 1	−3.7[b]	−3.4[c]
		Intervention 2	−4.9[b]	−4.6[c]
		Fibre	grams	
		Control	+2.2[b]	
		Intervention 1	+3.7[b]	+1.5
		Intervention 2	+5.5[b]	+3.3[c]
Tucker, Harris and Martin (1996)	12 weeks = end of intervention	Daily intake of		
		Energy	kcal	
		Control	−85	
		Intervention	−225[d]	−132
		Fat	% energy	
		Control	(+1)	
		Intervention	−4.5[d]	−3.4[c]
		Carbohydrate	% energy	
		Control	(−0.7)	
		Intervention	+4.2[d]	+3.3[c]

[a] Result in brackets indicates direction opposite to desired
[b] Not possible to assess statistical significance of before–after changes
[c] $p < 0.05$ for between-group difference
[d] $p < 0.05$ for change from baseline

Intake of fat

Three studies report data on this outcome – Brown, Lee and Oyomopito, Cox et al. and Tucker, Harris and Martin. Brown, Lee and Oyomopito report a statistically significant improvement in 'fat habit' scores in the intervention group, maintained for further 12-week follow-up, and a small, statistically non-significant, improvement in the control group, with the difference between the groups reaching statistical significance. It is difficult to assess what the change in these scores means in practice.

Cox et al. demonstrate greater reductions in the two intervention groups than control group at the end of the trial intervention period, the differences reaching statistical significance. The extent of the reductions are small to moderate but the baseline levels are not reported; the reductions may be worthwhile in practice if they are sustained.

Tucker, Harris and Martin demonstrate a reduction in fat intakes in the intervention group but not in the control group and the difference between the groups at the end of the trial is statistically significant and probably worthwhile in practice.

Intake of carbohydrate
Only Tucker, Harris and Martin report on this outcome directly. They indicate a statistically significant increase in intake in the intervention group and a slight, statistically non-significant reduction in the control group, the between-group difference being statistically significant. These results are consistent with the reported changes in fat intake.

Intake of fibre
Only Cox *et al.* report on this outcome, demonstrating a statistically significant but fairly small improvement in the 'EC' group, and a smaller, statistically non-significant improvement in the 'E' group, compared with controls. All three groups showed improvements in desired direction but it is not possible to calculate the statistical significance of the change compared with baseline within the groups.

Intake of energy
Cox *et al.* report small increases in energy intake in all three groups, with no statistically significant differences between the three groups. It is possible that the inclusion of some pregnant women in the study has contributed to this finding.

Tucker, Harris and Martin demonstrate small reductions in energy intake in control and intervention groups, and although the before–after difference in the intervention group is statistically significant, there is no statistically significant difference between the absolute levels at the end of the intervention.

Other
Johnson, Howell and Molloy demonstrated statistically significantly improved dietary intakes in intervention mothers compared with control mothers, at the end of the one-year intervention period. The extent of the improvement is impossible to assess because mean values for food items or nutrients are not reported.

The study by Brown, Lee and Oyomopito demonstrated that, compared with the control group, the intervention group showed statistically significant improvements in some anthropometric measurements, total cholesterol: HDL-C ratio (not reported here) and fitness indicators at the end of the intervention period. However, only the improvement in anthropometric measurements and the fitness indicators persisted until the 12-week follow-up.

In the study by Tucker, Harris and Martin, no differences were observed in protein or energy intake, or in anthropometric measurements.

Women who are pregnant – details of interventions and evaluations

With the exception of Anderson, Campbell and Shepherd, 1995, the interventions aimed at pregnant women (Sweeney et al., 1985; Kafatos, Vlachonikolis and Codrington, 1989; Villar et al., 1992; Belizán et al., 1995) all had the aim of improving pregnancy outcomes (primarily the incidence of low birthweight) by encouraging appropriate weight gain through pregnancy (see Table 6). These interventions all had an educational and counselling component and involved regular meetings from around the second trimester of pregnancy through to term, either in the clinic or at home visits. The participants were largely high-risk on the basis of past obstetric history or low socioeconomic status.

Table 6: Summary of rigorously evaluated interventions targeted at pregnant women

Study (in order of publication)	Type of intervention	How the intervention was delivered
Sweeney et al. (1985)	Education/counselling	Dietary counselling by dietitian enhanced by motivational video throughout pregnancy (ante-natal clinic)
Kafatos, Vlachonikolis and Codrington (1989)	Education/counselling	Dietary counselling by health worker throughout pregnancy (home visits)
Villar et al. (1992)/ Belizán et al. (1995)	Education/counselling/ psychosocial support	General support and counselling by health/ social worker throughout pregnancy (home visits)
Anderson, Campbell and Shepherd (1995)	Education	Information packs on nutrition at booking and mailed with personalised letter at 26 weeks gestation (ante-natal clinic/mailing)

Anderson's study, in contrast, evaluated an educational intervention which was targeted at improving healthy eating generally and which was not designed to improve pregnancy outcomes as a primary objective.

Details of individual reports

Sweeney, C, Smith, H, Foster, J C, Place, J C, Specht, J, Kochenour, N K and Prater, B M.
Effects of a nutrition intervention program during pregnancy: maternal data Phases 1 and 2.
Journal of Nurse Midwifery 1985; **30**:149–58.

This reports the results of a US RCT in which a clinic-based intervention to improve diet and weight gain in pregnancy, and so improve pregnancy outcomes, was assessed. The mean age of the subjects was 23 years and some of them were WIC enrollees. The intervention group received individual 'prescriptions' for protein and energy intake every 2–4 weeks from around 20 weeks' gestation to term and received explanation and 'counselling' from a dietitian; the intervention also included a one-off showing of a specially designed motivational video. The control group had their diets assessed in the same way as the intervention group, but the dietitian did not communicate a prescription to them, they were not 'counselled' and they watched a control video. The rationale for this study was to test the Higgins' intervention method for nutritional rehabilitation during pregnancy (Higgins, 1976), a system of nutritional assessment, prescription and counselling developed over a period of time in Montreal. The interest of the authors is the effect of the intervention on low birthweight and infant health and details of counselling aspects of the intervention are very limited.

Outcomes were assessed in terms of consumption (> 85%) of the prescribed dietary intake, as assessed by 7-day recall by interview and grocery purchase/household food intake cross-check, and weight gain during pregnancy.

Many important methodological points were not reported and the study was described by the authors as a pilot. The comparison is of the effect of explaining the prescription/nutrition counselling plus the motivational video with the effect of having a prescription assessed but not communicated plus the control video. It would not be possible to attribute any effects to one or other of these components separately without further investigation. The authors also acknowledge that the study was limited by insufficient power. Collection of data on nutrition outcomes appeared to be carried out by observers who were aware of the allocation status of the participants and the data collection methods were variable. This introduces a considerable potential for bias in favour of the intervention.

Kafatos, A G, Vlachonikolis, I G and Codrington, C A.
Nutrition during pregnancy: the effects of an educational intervention program in Greece.
American Journal of Clinical Nutrition 1989; **50**:970–9.

This reports an RCT conducted in Greece which aimed to improve maternal diet and weight gain in pregnancy, and so improve pregnancy outcomes. The participants were pregnant women, mean age 23 years, with > 70% from low SES backgrounds. The intervention was delivered in the home setting and consisted of 1:1 education ('instruction')/ counselling by a health professional 2-weekly from enrolment to delivery. No further details are given on how this intervention was developed or a theoretical framework, although it is stated that the nurses at the intervention clinics received 'intensive training'. No details are given regarding the control group, and it is assumed that they contributed data only.

Intakes of the main nutrients, vitamins and iron were assessed at several points throughout pregnancy in a proportion of participants using 24-hour recall and weighed intakes and weight gain in pregnancy was calculated.

Despite the large sample size, questions remain over baseline comparability of groups, blinding, follow-up and lack of control intervention. The cluster randomisation (by clinic) was not taken into account in analysis (by individual), with the effect that statistical tests are likely to over-estimate statistical significance (Buck and Donner, 1982; Donner, Birkett and Buck, 1981; Donner and Donald, 1987; Whiting-O'Keefe, Henke and Simborg, 1984).

Villar, J, Farnot, U, Barros, F, Victora, C, Langer, A and Belizán, J M.
A randomized trial of psychosocial support during high-risk pregnancies.
New England Journal of Medicine 1992; **327**:1266–71.

Belizán, J M, Barros, F, Langer, A, Farnot, U, Victora, C and Villar, J.
Impact of health education during pregnancy on behavior and utilization of health resources.
American Journal of Obstetrics and Gynecology 1995; **173**:894–9.

Taken together, these papers report the methodology and results of a large international RCT conducted in Argentina, Brazil, Cuba and Mexico. The aim of the intervention was to improve pregnancy outcomes in women at high risk of delivering an infant of low birthweight. The intervention comprised three components (Langer *et al.*, 1993), reinforcement of the pregnant woman's social network and emotional support; improvement in her knowledge about pregnancy and delivery; and reinforcement of adequate utilisation of health services. The rationale was based on previous published literature that suggested that women with lower psychological distress, better knowledge about pregnancy and better use of health services have better outcomes. The educational component of the intervention was delivered during 4–6 home visits by a social or health care professional through pregnancy; a standard manual of operations was developed following ethnographic studies in each trial site, and the home visitors developed a flexible individual plan for each participant in conjunction with the study supervisor, after the initial home visit. The home visitors provided one-to-one advice, encouragement and 'emotional support' to the participants, who were also given a poster/booklet and open access to a special patient support office and hotline. The control group received routine prenatal care only. The mean age of the participants was 24.4 years.

The primary outcomes of this trial related to pregnancy, but data were also collected on 'improvement in diet' as assessed by a dietitian on the basis of interview data at 36 weeks gestation. Use of iron or folate supplements was also ascertained by an independent interviewer at 36 weeks gestation.

This was a rigorous trial from the point of view of primary outcomes of interest (obstetric) but the nutrition outcome measures were extremely limited and the validity of the assessment tools is unclear.

Anderson, A S, Campbell, D M and Shepherd, R.
The influence of dietary advice on nutrient intake during pregnancy. *British Journal of Nutrition* 1995; **73**:163–77.

This paper reported a UK clinic-based RCT where the intervention aimed to alter nutrition knowledge, attitudes and behaviour. The development of the intervention and its evaluation followed formative research surveys in the study population and piloting of the data gathering instruments. The underlying rationale was to capitalise on pregnancy as a period when women may be more ready to change health behaviour. The intervention was not designed to alter pregnancy outcomes. The mean age of the participants was 26 years and 30 per cent were from non-manual RG classes. The intervention group received information packs on nutrition at their booking appointment and at 26 weeks gestation, the second pack accompanied by a personalised letter from a named doctor. The control group received the general pregnancy health guide given to all pregnant women booking at that clinic (including women in the intervention group).

Assessment tools were developed using the framework described by Ajzen and Fishbein (Ajzen and Fishbein, 1980) and encompassed knowledge, attitudes and behaviour. Nutrition knowledge was assessed by a questionnaire developed for the study, with a score calculated for knowledge of nutrition terms, theoretical principles and practical applications. Attitude scores were calculated from questions in the same questionnaire. Nutrient intakes were calculated from 4-day diary records, prospectively recorded.

The evaluation of the intervention was fairly rigorous although there was potential for contamination between groups, which would tend to dilute any effect of the intervention. The follow-up rate for the two groups was over 80 per cent for the questionnaires but fell below 70 per cent for the dietary diaries; however, the attrition and reasons for drop-out were similar across the two groups. Although no sample size calculations were reported the study was certainly powerful enough to detect important differences in dietary intakes between the groups. No baseline nutrition intake data were provided for the two groups so it is not possible to assess within-group before–after changes.

Pregnant women – details of outcomes

Most of the studies reported post-test data only, so it is not possible to comment on before–after changes in the indicators for control and intervention groups for most of the outcomes.

Only Anderson, Campbell and Shepherd assessed knowledge and attitudes as outcomes. They demonstrated a small but statistically significant difference between the intervention and control groups in the total knowledge score (Table 7). On average, this would amount to improving a total knowledge score from 10/19 to 11/19. This improvement was almost entirely accounted for by an improvement in the 'practical application' component, towards which the assessment tool was weighted, where the difference between the intervention and control groups amounted to 0.8/11 (see Appendix G for further details).

Details of the attitude scores are given in Appendix G, with the 'behavioural intention' component included in Table 7. For each component the intervention group scored more highly than the control group but the differences were slight and statistically non-significant.

Table 7: Improvement in key nutrition outcomes in pregnant women

Study	Timing of assessment	Extent of change within group following intervention between groups		Absolute difference following intervention
Knowledge				
Anderson, Campbell and Shepherd (1995)	30 weeks' gestation	Total score (maximum possible = 19) Control Intervention	Not estimable	+0.9[a]
Attitudes				
Anderson, Campbell and Shepherd (1995)	30 weeks' gestation	Behavioural intention score (maximum possible = +3) Control Intervention	Not estimable	+0.1
Behaviour				
Villar et al. (1992), Belizán et al. (1995)	36 weeks' gestation	Percentage reporting improvement in diet Control Intervention	+8.9[b] 11.8[b]	+0.3
Anderson Campbell and Shepherd (1995)	30 weeks' gestation	Daily intake of Energy Control Intervention	kJ Not estimable	−84
		Fat Control Intervention	% energy Not estimable	−0.8
		Carbohydrate Control Intervention	% energy Not estimable	+0.3
		Fibre Control Intervention	grams Not estimable	+0.9
Sweeney et al. (1985)	During intervention	Daily intake of Energy Control Intervention	kcal Not estimable	+189
Kafatos, Vlachonikolis and Codrington (1989)	During intervention	Daily intake of Energy Control Intervention	kcal Not estimable	(point estimate not reported – best estimate of range of difference) +224–418[e]

[a] $p < 0.05$ for between-group difference [b] $p < 0.05$ for change from baseline [c] Statistical significance not reported because of unit of analysis error

Intake of fat

Both Anderson, Campbell and Shepherd and Kafatos, Vlachonikolis and Codrington assessed this outcome. Anderson and colleagues' results favour the intervention but the difference was very small and not statistically significant. Kafatos and colleagues demonstrated differences in this outcome of around 10 g per day between intervention and control groups from 22 weeks to term. It was not possible to report these data here directly as they are presented in graphical form only, and they are subject to a unit of analysis error.

Intake of carbohydrate

Both Anderson, Campbell and Shepherd and Kafatos, Vlachonikolis and Codrington assessed this outcome. Again, Anderson and colleagues' results favour the intervention but the difference was very small and not statistically significant. Kafatos and colleagues demonstrated differences of around 30–60 g per day between intervention and control groups after 29 weeks' gestation but baseline differences of about 30 g per day between groups should be noted. It was not possible to report these data here directly as they are presented in graphical form only and they are subject to a unit of analysis error.

Intake of fibre

Only Anderson, Campbell and Shepherd report on this outcome; they demonstrated small but not statistically significant changes.

Energy

Three reports present data on this outcome: Anderson, Campbell and Shepherd; Kafatos, Vlachonikolis and Codrington; and Sweeney *et al.* Anderson and colleagues again demonstrate only a small difference between the intervention and control groups, in favour of the intervention, but not reaching statistical significance. Kafatos and colleagues demonstrated differences between groups of about 200 or more kcal per day, throughout the data collection period, in favour of the intervention group. The baseline difference between groups of about 150 kcal per day should be noted. Sweeney *et al.* report a difference of +189 kcal per day in the intervention group, compared with the control group, but this difference did not reach statistical significance.

Other

Villar *et al.* did not report nutrient intakes directly, but presented categorical data on the proportion of participants who had 'improved' their diet. Both control and intervention groups showed a statistically significant improvement in this indicator over the course of the trial but the difference between the groups at the end of the trial was not statistically significant.

Brief details of other interventions targeted at women of childbearing age and pregnant women

Each of the following interventions was excluded from the review on the basis of scope or methodology. However, together they illustrate and exemplify the range of intervention types encountered during the review and each approach might merit formal evaluation using a rigorous design.

Cook it! (A McQueen, personal communication – see Appendix B) This intervention aimed to promote low-cost healthy cooking in the community. It was developed by the Health Promotion Agency for Northern Ireland and used pre-existing groups (mother and toddler groups) as a conduit to the whole family in areas with a high proportion of low-income residents.

Kumanyika, S K and Charleston, J B.
Lose weight and win: a church-based weight loss program for blood pressure control among black women.
Patient Education and Counseling 1992; **19**:19–32.

This US study involved church-going women (aged 18–81) of a particular ethnic group predisposed to a diet-related illness; it consisted of an eight-week exercise and counselling programme. Using an existing group such as this (or the one described above) provides a social element to the intervention and provides participants with a reference group (i.e. what one can achieve compared to one's peers) and it could be translated to the UK.

Larsson, I and Lissner, L.
The Green Keyhole nutritional campaign in Sweden: do women with more knowledge have better dietary practices?
European Journal of Clinical Nutrition 1996; **50**:323–8.

This Swedish study aimed to ascertain whether women changed their purchasing behaviour in response to a national food marking intervention, which labelled low-fat and high-fibre foods with a 'Green Keyhole' symbol. The authors suggest that 'it is likely that the keyhole has provided an important stimulus for food manufacturers to develop reduced fat and enriched fibre products'. The use of a symbol to promote healthy foods is simple and does not depend on the literacy or education level of the consumer. There are many parallels in the UK but it is unclear whether they lead to improved diet.

Quinn, T J and Jenkins, M.
Nutritional profiles of selected college females in a 15-week exercise and
weight control class.
Health Values 1991; **15**:34–41.

This US uncontrolled before-and-after study involved students receiving
an intervention as part of their course work. They received education
(information on diet, food labelling, etc.), exercise instruction, self-
directed learning as well as their own nutritional profile with individual
recommendations. Positive peer pressure to motivate participants was
built in through logging of exercise which needed to be signed by two
fellow students.

Simkin-Silverman, L, Wing, R and Hansen, D H.
Prevention of cardiovascular risk factor elevations in healthy
premenopausal women.
Preventive Medicine 1995; **24**:509–17.

This intervention was targeted at reducing cardiovascular risk factors in
women approaching the menopause and involved a fairly intensive
behavioural change intervention through group work. The intervention
included problem-solving exercise, relapse prevention, and stimulus
control techniques. The findings suggested the approach was effective
within the timescale studied. As in all group programmes there is the
motivational effect of positive peer pressure, but the more widespread
application might be limited by the requirement for input by specialised
staff.

5. Discussion

The aim of this review was to identify effective interventions for promoting healthier diet in women of childbearing age and pregnant women. Considering how to address this aim led us to identify immediately a number of issues which went to the heart of the approach and methods we adopted. We adopted the notion of 'effectiveness' in line with current thinking in health services and clinical research – an effective intervention is one which brings about a measurable change in a desired outcome, and in which the change can be attributed with some confidence to the intervention and not to some external factor, for example background changes in society, or the well-known effect of just taking part in a research study (the so-called 'Hawthorne effect'). Because many researchers, though well-intentioned, may be less than disinterested investigators, assessing effectiveness as defined above requires adherence to widely accepted and promulgated methodological principles (Monsen and Cheney, 1988; Sackett, Haynes and Tugwell, 1985); these are designed to minimise the inherent bias which tends to produce exaggerated effect sizes of interventions, to ensure that useful effects are not missed because studies have too few participants, and to produce results which can be extrapolated beyond the immediate population in which the research took place.

These characteristics describe pragmatic, rigorous evaluation which is designed to answer the question 'how effective is this intervention when put into practice?' However, a well-designed evaluation cannot compensate for an *intervention* that is poorly designed or thought out; the development of potentially effective interventions in the field of health promotion depends on effective formative research to uncover general concepts and principles, frameworks to illuminate how such principles might be translated into interventions and pilot testing of potential interventions in the target populations of interest. While details of the different interventions reviewed have been extracted, it was not possible within the timescale of this review to comment in detail on this aspect of research.

Having set out our stall as above, we therefore restricted the review to evaluative studies based on experimental or quasi-experimental designs (Sackett, Haynes and Tugwell, 1985), meaning randomised controlled trials (RCTs) and controlled, non-randomised studies (controlled before and after (CBA) studies and interrupted time series analysis (ITS) studies) (Cook and Campbell, 1979). We have drawn a distinction between the notion of 'efficacy', where a 'clinical' effect is demonstrated under highly controlled conditions (for example in a 'laboratory'-type environment) and 'effectiveness', which implies a useful change in a health outcome when an intervention is implemented in situations resembling real life, where compliance, for example, may be more difficult to ensure. Our review concentrates on evaluations which are conducted in field settings and which, it is hoped, have some external validity (generalisability). Because of the limited number of reports identified, however, we were flexible in our inclusion criteria and were inclusive rather than exclusive of some reports where the target population did not fit strictly within our definitions (for example the Latin American trial reported by Villar and colleagues (1992), the work by Brown, Lee and Oyomopito (1996) in Greek–Australian women). However, we excluded a number of studies where the aim of the intervention was weight management in overweight subjects, and not healthy eating per se or where the aim was to assess *the effect of* supplementation with vitamins and other nutrients. However, our criteria did not exclude reports of interventions designed to prevent obesity in non-obese subjects (of which we found none with this specific intention), or reports of interventions *to encourage women to consume* appropriate recommended supplementation, for example folic acid supplements (the work by, for example, Sweeney et al. (1985) could be considered in this category).

The validity of a review such as this should be judged by whether most or all relevant studies are likely to have been identified, whether they have been appropriately appraised, and whether the overall conclusions appear to be consistent with the material reviewed. This review identified disappointingly few evaluations fulfilling the inclusion criteria. This is unlikely to be because the search was not wide enough as a large number of electronic bibliographic databases were searched and many experts were contacted. While it is possible that a greater emphasis on locating reports contained within the 'grey' literature might have identified some extra useful studies it is unlikely that many of sufficient rigour would have been picked up. Our experience with hand-searching specialist health promotion journals was that it did not yield studies fulfilling the inclusion criteria; this has also been our experience in conducting another, separate review in the field of nutrition and health behaviour and provides some reassurance that important published studies were unlikely to have been missed. We also note the experience of Smith et al. (1997), who surveyed six public health journals using manual searching and found that 14 per cent of the 603 studies were interventions, and only four per cent were RCTs. They concluded that of those not using randomisation, 42 per cent could have, and that RCTs were underused; they took this as an indication of a lack of methodological rigour (and possibly understanding) in research in community health and it is likely that the same applies to evaluation in health promotion.

What is of more concern is the possibility that relevant unpublished work remains unidentified, and that papers published in languages other than English were specifically excluded. Unpublished trials are more likely than published trial to have null results; if we were able to identify and include such trials then the most likely effect would be to dilute any overall positive effects and so weaken the evidence of effectiveness. All other things being equal, trials published in non-English languages are no more likely or unlikely to be positive or null than those published in English – in effect, their (potential) exclusion lessens the 'power' of the review, but should have little effect on qualitative conclusions about effectiveness.

The identification of only nine relevant trials in total is disappointing, as is the fairly poor quality of many of these studies, but this is by no means uncommon in the field of systematic reviews in health services research. We can only conclude that very few reliable evaluations in this field have been conducted, despite the wealth of observational data. No articles were identified which evaluated wider health promotion interventions such as media campaigns or community development in a rigorous manner in a target population of interest to this review.

The interventions in women of childbearing age were all delivered in community settings and most of them had an educational component, but they were diverse in their aims, how they were delivered and underlying conceptual frameworks. In none of the reports was preparation for pregnancy or motherhood identified as a specific reason for improving diet. Taken together, they provide little data on the extent to which nutritional knowledge is improved, but suggest that it is possible to promote healthier eating, particularly lower fat intakes, for the duration of the interventions. As no long-term follow-up data are provided it is not possible to comment whether the effects are likely to be sustained.

Three out of the four interventions in pregnant women had the aim of improving pregnancy outcomes in women who were at some obstetric risk, for example of producing a baby of low birthweight. Only Anderson and colleagues (1995) designed an intervention to promote healthy eating 'for life', targeting pregnant women because they might be more susceptible to health education messages than the general population. All of the interventions had an educational component; in the three pregnancy-outcome oriented studies this was supplemented by individual counselling in the clinic setting (Sweeney et al., 1985) or at home (Kafatos, Vlachonikolis and Codrington, 1989) or was delivered as part of a wider effort at providing psychosocial support throughout pregnancy (Villar et al., 1992). The intervention tested by Anderson and colleagues (1995) was designed after a period of formative research and was designed to improve knowledge and promote positive attitudes and behaviour, but was not mediated by a health professional in person.

Anderson and Kafatos and colleagues produced findings which suggest that it is possible to achieve improvement in diets in pregnant women, although the extent of the improvements is marginal in the former and much more impressive in the latter study. This might reflect the enhancing effect of an individual who acts as an adviser, supporter and counsellor, but it may also be due, in part, to an exaggeration of the true effect in the study by Kafatos and colleagues, which was marred by a unit of analysis error and other potential biases. Sweeney's results are limited by the aims of the trial – to encourage eating to a 'prescription' in order to improve maternal weight gain – and have limited generalisability. The study by Villar and colleagues demonstrates that an improvement in diet in pregnancy is possible, but no specific information is provided on what is meant by an 'improvement' and they fail to demonstrate that this is the result of their intervention, rather than what would have occurred without intervention or as a result of the Hawthorne effect.

Anderson and colleagues demonstrated small but positive differences in knowledge and attitudes in the participants receiving their intervention but this was not translated into worthwhile behavioural change. This is consistent with the findings of Goode et al. (1994) who reported a survey of 420 adults, and in-depth interviews with 75, regarding how dietary choices are made in the context of the social, cultural and economic situation. They express a view that, for their survey population, there were high levels of awareness of healthy eating campaigns but many did not make dietary changes in line with government recommendations. Goode and colleagues argue that this 'confirms the need for explanations other than those which simply rest on the idea of a rational response to information'. There are a number of well recognised barriers to behavioural change in general and dietary change in particular, such as cost, availability, access, family eating patterns, support from others, and personal belief in the ability to change (self efficacy).

Even if the results of the studies are credible, caution must be exercised before recommending the general implementation of their findings. Often behavioural change is reported in health promotion campaigns during and shortly after the running of the programme, but long-term sustained change is far less likely to be reported (Edwards, Acock and Johnson, 1985; Ernst et al., 1986).

Conclusions

Despite a comprehensive literature search, only relatively few rigorous evaluations of interventions to promote healthy eating in the target population were identified. Around three times as many studies evaluating interventions were excluded than included, mainly because they were uncontrolled or had uninterpretable outcome data. This suggests that there is need for researchers evaluating health promotion initiatives to improve their understanding of evaluative research techniques, as a complement to observational and qualitative research methods which are more directly relevant to the development of potential new interventions than to the assessment of their effectiveness.

The interventions in women of childbearing age were diverse and appeared to suggest that, in general, it is possible to improve the nutrition knowledge of women of childbearing age and to improve diets (particularly fat intake) while interventions are being delivered. However, it is not possible to recommend, without reservation, the general implementation of the interventions identified here, because they were generally evaluated insufficiently rigorously and did not include evidence of the sustainability of the changes.

Taken together, it is difficult to determine whether or not the interventions in pregnant women, which were targeted at improving pregnancy outcomes, were worthwhile, because of limitations in the evaluation methodologies. The largest effect sizes were observed in a study in which the findings are likely to be exaggerated because of methodological flaws and unlikely to be generalisable to the UK population. These interventions all involved counselling, of varying intensity, by a trained professional throughout pregnancy. A single study in pregnant women stood out because the intervention did not involve one-to-one counselling (and therefore was likely to be cheaper than the others), and was targeted at healthy eating as an end in itself; this intervention was evaluated fairly rigorously and produced small, generally null, results in terms of knowledge, attitudes and nutrition behaviour.

Future research in this area should concentrate on establishing the rationale for dietary counselling interventions in pregnancy – both their purpose and the groups of women who might benefit most. Intervention studies in this area could and should adhere to the general principles of rigorous study design, particularly in relation to observer blinding and the use of valid and reliable instruments and include an assessment of the long-term nutrition outcomes, beyond the delivery of a healthy baby.

The overwhelming need is for carefully designed, pragmatic trials of sufficient size to produce findings which can be confidently extrapolated to the wider population.

Appendices

Appendix A. Details of methodology

Scope and approach of the review

The review focused on interventions to promote improvements in dietary behaviour in free-living women of childbearing age or pregnant women. We adopted a definition of 'healthy eating' appropriate to the time period in which relevant reports were being published as dictated by the timescale of the review (i.e. from the early 1980s onward).

We adopted the following definition of 'health promotion': 'any planned measure which promotes health or prevents disease, disability and premature death' (Whitehead, 1991). This encompasses health education, counselling, changes in environment and changes in policy. All interventions aimed at improving diet were included, irrespective of whether or not this was the investigators' explicit or implicit primary goal.

The methods of review were based upon those used by the Cochrane Collaboration and the Centre for Reviews and Dissemination (NHS Centre for Reviews and Dissemination, 1996).

Inclusion of studies
Inclusion criteria
Studies which fulfilled the following criteria were eligible for inclusion in the systematic review:

Target population
Studies which targeted free-living women of childbearing age and/or pregnant women. By free-living we mean not living permanently in institutions, for example prison or hospital. Specifically excluded were studies targeting women at clinically-defined high risk of diet-related disease, for example diabetic women, malnourished women. We anticipated that there may be very few published reports of evaluations targeting women of childbearing age specifically, so we widened the scope of the search to include studies with the following types of participants:

- women recruited because they are of childbearing age
- women of childbearing age (15–45 or thereabouts if not otherwise specified) recruited for other or unspecified reasons

women of childbearing age recruited as part of a study of a wider population of adult women only (i.e. with a proportion of participants older than childbearing age, but not including males). Where possible, results specific to the subgroup of women with childbearing age were sought.

Study design
Studies in which the design was a randomised controlled trial, controlled before and after study, or an interrupted time series analysis.

Intervention
Studies which described interventions designed to promote a 'healthier' diet. Given the probable variation in the precise dietary objectives targeted in different intervention studies, we defined as 'healthy eating' any target outcome broadly in line with the National Advisory Committee on Nutrition Education's (NACNE) 1983 recommendations (NACNE, 1983):

(a) total fat intake of 115 g or less per day (34% of total energy) (i.e. reduction)
(b) an average intake of saturated fatty acids of 50 g or less per day (15% of total energy) (i.e. reduction)
(c) an average intake of polyunsaturated fatty acids of 18 g or more per day (5% of total energy) (i.e. increase)
(d) an intake of less than 30 g of sucrose per day (12% of total energy) (i.e. reduction in sugar intake) (i.e. reduction)
(e) maintenance of energy intake through low-fat foods, particularly bread, potatoes, fruit and vegetables (i.e. increase)
(f) an intake of 25 g or more of dietary fibre per day (i.e. increase)
(g) an intake of 1 g or less of salt per day (i.e. reduction).

Studies were included if they targeted one or more of these factors, whatever methods were used.

Outcomes
Studies which used outcome indicators relevant to the intervention which included and presented interpretable results.

Timescale
Studies published between 1985 and the time the review was conducted.

Language
Only studies published in the English language were included.

Identification of studies
Development of search strategy for identification of studies for inclusion

The first search strategies were developed on MEDLINE using the OVID software interface. MEDLINE was used extensively in the early stages of the study to identify appropriate subject headings, key words and phrases. Search terms were built up by investigating Medical Subject Headings (MeSH) using the MeSH tree, scope notes and Permuted Index. These terms were then organised into four distinct sections.

(a) study design – this section was based upon the standard strategy used by the Cochrane Collaboration Review Groups; it was modified and expanded to include terms for intervention studies
(b) health promotion and health education
(c) nutrition and dietary
(d) pregnancy and childbearing age.

The general format consisted of different combinations of study design, health promotion and nutrition terms, with specific pregnancy/childbearing age terms added to focus the search. Initial searches were sensitive rather than specific.

Non-MEDLINE strategies

Separate strategies were developed for each individual electronic database. This was necessary primarily because of different indexing systems and differences in terminology and phraseology. The search strategies developed on MEDLINE were, however, eligible to run on CINAHL and the Cochrane Library database. Thus there were a large number of searches conducted with a wide variety of relevant terms employed.

Electronic databases

The following list of electronic databases was systematically searched for eligible studies. Databases were accessed either on compact disk format or via online servers:

ASSIA+ (Abstracts in Social Medicine, CD-ROM)
Centre for Pregnancy and Nutrition, Sheffield (internal database search)
CINAHL (Cumulative Index of Nursing and Allied Health, CD-ROM)
Cochrane Library (1997 CD-ROM issue 2, incorporating Cochrane Database of Systematic Reviews, Database of Reviews of Effectiveness, Cochrane Review Methodology Database, Cochrane Controlled Trials Register)
CRIB (Current Research in Britain, CD-ROM)
ERIC (Education Research)
EDINA Biosis (Edinburgh Data and Information Access, online)
EMBASE (electronic version of Excerpta Medica)
HEBS (Health Education Board for Scotland, CD-ROM)

MEDLINE (electronic version of Index Medicus, online)
MIDIRS (Midwives Information and Resource Service database search)
National Childbirth Trust (via NCT library)
PsycLIT (American Psychological Association, CD-ROM)
SIGLE (Sources in Grey Literature Europe, CD-ROM)
Sociofile (CD-ROM)
Science Citation Index (online)
Social Science Citation Index (online)
UNICORN (Health Education Authority internal database).

Other methods of identifying studies for inclusion
Reference lists of selected articles

The reference lists of review articles, narrative articles, studies eligible for inclusion and relevant book chapters on the topics of interest were checked for eligible references:

Journal of Nutrition Education 1985 special edition (a meta-analysis and synthesis of nutrition education research, 1985)
HEA Coronary Prevention Group 1993 (HEA, 1993)
Andrien (1994)
Cucherat and Boissel (1993)
Liedekerken *et al.* (1990)
Boyd and Windsor (1993)
Trouba, Okereke and Splett (1991)
Fugate Woods (1991)
A guide to effective care in pregnancy and childbirth (Chalmers, Enkin and Keirse, 1989)
Health Promotion Library Scotland Bulletin 1993–96
Health Lines (includes Current Awareness Bulletin) 1993–96
Current Research in Britain 10th edition
BDA list of members' research interests
Quality assessment in health promotion and health education: proceedings of Third European Conference on Effectiveness, 1996 (Italy)
Proceedings of Fifth Health Services Research Conference, 1993 (The Netherlands).

Hand-searching

It has been reported by experienced researchers that electronic bibliographic databases miss a significant proportion of randomised controlled trials because of inconsistent indexing. A number of journals were identified through consultation with experts as the most likely to yield relevant reports and hand-searched to identify eligible studies.

American Journal of Public Health	1985–96
British Journal of Nutrition	1985–96
Evaluation Review	1992–96
(incomplete)	

Health Education Quarterly	1995 v.22
Health Education Research	1993–96
Health Promotion International	1992–96
Health Promotion Journal of Australia (incomplete)	1991–96
American Dietetic Association Journal	1985–95
Journal of Human Nutrition and Dietetics	1987–94
Journal of Nutrition Education (incomplete)	1985–96
Nutrition and Health	1986–96
Preventive Medicine (incomplete)	1985–96
Proceedings of the Nutrition Society	1985–96

Contact with specialist agencies and experts in the field

A number of health promotion, health education and specialist libraries and agencies were contacted for information. The Health Promotion Library Scotland and the Health Education Authority conducted electronic searches on internal databases. Requests for information were sent to a number of health promotion and nutrition experts throughout the United Kingdom. An electronic mail request for information was circulated on health promotion and nutrition mailbases. Appendix B lists the individuals and organisations who responded to requests for information.

Identification of studies and data management

All electronically-derived study titles and abstracts were read to assess relevance and potential for inclusion. All potential trials were electronically imported or manually entered into a reference manager software package (Reference Manager, Professional Edition (Research Information Systems, 1995)). Studies were then organised into two databases, one for women of childbearing age and one for pregnant women.

Databases were then searched in greater detail and requests for hard copies of potential trials for inclusion were made. Hard copies of references were obtained from local libraries, distant collections using the University of Aberdeen inter-library loan system, personal collections and personal requests to authors.

Review of studies
Data extraction forms

Four standardised data extraction forms were designed, piloted and developed by the research team (Appendix C). These forms were based upon those developed by the Cochrane Collaboration on Effective Professional Practice (Bero *et al.*, 1996a, 1996b).

(a) *Data extraction form – inclusion criteria and basic study details*
   This form was completed for all studies thought to fulfil the inclusion criteria. This form comprised questions relating to scope,

study design, interpretability and intervention. If a study failed to fulfil these criteria, it was excluded from the review. Those which did fulfil the criteria were then further assessed using one of the three data extraction forms relating to study design.

(b) *Data extraction form – randomised controlled trials*
Each study of randomised controlled trial design was independently assessed by two reviewers for methodological quality. Details of participants, intervention and outcomes were recorded in a standardised format on the data extraction form.

(c) *Data extraction form – controlled before and after studies*
Each controlled before-and-after study was independently assessed by two reviewers for methodological quality. Details of participants, intervention and outcomes were recorded in a standardised format on the data extraction form.

(d) *Data extraction form – interrupted time series studies*
Each interrupted time series study was independently assessed by two reviewers for methodological quality. Details of participants, intervention and outcomes were recorded in a standardised format on the data extraction form.

Assessing the quality of evidence of the studies
A hierarchy of evidence was adopted, namely randomised controlled trials (RCTs), controlled before-and-after studies (CBAs) and interrupted time series analyses (ITSs), in descending order of robustness. In practice, no interrupted time series studies were identified and so the review contains only randomised and non-randomised trials with concurrent control groups.

For RCTs and CBAs, the following criteria were used to judge quality:

1. The units of allocation and analysis were the same (i.e. the analysis was based on the same 'units', for example individuals or groups, which were originally allocated to the intervention and control groups).
2. Power calculations were reported (i.e. the study had sufficient power to detect clinically important effects as statistically significant).
3. There was adequate follow-up (> 80 per cent) of study subjects (i.e. protection against exclusion bias).
4. There was evidence of blinded assessment of primary outcome(s) (i.e. protection against detection bias).
5. The intervention and control groups appeared comparable for main outcome measures at baseline.
6. There was evidence of protection against contamination (i.e. behaviour in control group was unlikely to have been influenced by exposure in some way to the intervention).

In addition, the following criterion was used for RCTs only:

7. There was evidence of concealment of allocation of subjects to intervention and control groups (i.e. protection against selection bias).

Process of reviewing studies

A half-day training workshop was developed by BJW and attended by the other reviewers (NB, AR, GMcN). The topics covered included: the rationale for the review, eligibility criteria, indicators of quality of study design, and the reviewing timetable and practicalities.

BJW acted as first reviewer for each study and the other three acted as independent second reviewer for a third of the articles each. Each candidate report identified by NB was allocated to each pair of reviewers, who each received a photocopy of the article along with a set of data extraction forms. The paired reviewers were responsible for the final allocation of reports to eligible and ineligible categories, by discussing disagreements if necessary. If they could not agree on the category of any report, it was passed on to a third reviewer for independent review and a final decision through discussion.

Data extraction and analysis
Type of participants

Included studies were subdivided according to whether they targeted pregnant women or women of childbearing age. If they targeted both they were reported in each category, if outcome data on the different types of participants were reported separately; otherwise they were allocated to the category appropriate for the largest proportion of participants.

Intervention type

Studies were categorised according to the nature of the reported intervention, and its duration. Where insufficient details were presented to be sure about the intervention type, a judgement was made as to the likely type of intervention by EVT and BJW.

Data extraction and analysis

Tables are presented separately for pregnant women and women of childbearing age. Data were extracted for the primary outcomes reported in each paper, in the three categories knowledge, attitudes, behaviour. Where a range of indicators of intake were reported, markers of fat, carbohydrate, fibre and energy intake were selected, along with biological markers such as serum or plasma cholesterol; anthropometric measures such as body mass index and % body fat were also included. For each study, baseline and post-intervention nutrition outcome data were extracted for all control and intervention groups, where possible.

Where outcomes were reported at different periods after the intervention, the last available measurement was extracted, so long as it applied to all control and intervention groups. BJW alone was responsible for extracting quantitative outcome data from all included studies.

Wherever possible, data on mean intakes were sought. Before–after differences in mean intake for each outcome were calculated for each control and intervention group and, if reporting was complete, statistical significance recorded (if reported appropriately in the source report) or calculated using Student's t-test (for paired samples if possible, otherwise unpaired). Where data on sample size or standard deviation were missing, mean values and within group differences were reported but statistical significance could not be calculated.

For any studies with a possible unit of analysis error (where cluster randomisation had been used but not taken into account in the original analysis), mean values and differences were reported but statistical testing was not performed or disregarded.

Between-group differences between control or baseline and each intervention group were also calculated and statistical significance calculated using unpaired Student's t-test, subject to the same proviso regarding unit of analysis above.

Where possible, categorical data were tested using the χ^2 test.

The heterogeneity of interventions, target groups, study designs and statistical techniques meant that full meta-analysis of the results was impossible.

Studies reporting interventions which were evaluated in an insufficiently rigorous manner are listed for completeness but were not fully reviewed or tabulated. However, a brief description is included of selected interventions which, in the judgement of the authors, might merit formal rigorous evaluation. It is emphasised that their effectiveness in pregnant women and women of childbearing age is unproven.

The WIC Program

We have reviewed separately reports of evaluations of the US Special Supplemental Food Program for Women, Infants and Children (the WIC Program), (Rush et al., 1988a–e). Very few of these reports fulfilled our methodological inclusion criteria and most of them focused on pregnancy outcomes (for example birthweight) rather than nutrition outcomes. However, we felt that a commentary would be useful both for completeness, and because of the importance and cost of this initiative. This is reported in Appendix D.

Appendix B. Organisations and individuals contacted

A list of key contacts and addresses for the organisations listed below is available from the authors.

Organisations
AHCPR Publications Clearinghouse
American Public Health Association Clearinghouse on Infant Feeding and Maternal Nutrition
British Dietetic Association
Centre for Pregnancy Nutrition
The Cochrane Collaboration on Effective Professional Practice (CCEPP), University of York
Forth Valley Health Board
Grampian Health Board
Grampian Health Promotions
Health Education Authority
Health Education Board Scotland
Health Promotion Wales
Highland Health Board
King's Fund Library and Information Service
Lothian Health Board
NHS Centre for Reviews and Dissemination
Northern Health and Social Services Board
Public Health Nutrition Discussion and Information Group [phnutr-l@u.washington.edu]
Shetland Health Board
SocHealth: The Health Sociology Electronic Mail Newsletter

Individuals
U Arens, British Nutrition Foundation
G Coburn, Oxford PHC
P Donnithorne, The National Childbirth Trust
W Doyle, Queen Elizabeth Hospital for Children
P Hunt, Oxfordshire
A McQueen, Health Promotion and Health Education Belfast
R Minnis, British Dietetic Association
S O'Meara, York University
M Rayner, University of Oxford
L Roe, University of Oxford
J Thomas, Kings College, University of London

Appendix C. The data extraction form

The data extraction form was designed to be completed in two stages. Sections 1 and 2 were completed for all candidate studies and were designed to assist the decision to include or exclude the study and to capture basic descriptive data on all interventions. Data were then extracted from studies fulfilling the inclusion criteria, using the appropriate version of Section 3, RCT or CBA. A section was also designed for interrupted time series studies, but as none was identified it is not reproduced here. Please note that the data extraction forms have been reproduced here in reduced form – full copies, including the ITS section, are obtainable on request by writing to:

Dr Brenda J Wilson
Department of Public Health
University of Aberdeen
Polwarth Building
Foresterhill
Aberdeen AB25 2ZD

Email: b.j.wilson@abdn.ac.uk

Main guidance

Sections 1 and 2

Section 1 of the standard data extraction form should be filled in by two independent reviewers to check inclusion/exclusion criteria.

Section 2 should be filled in for all studies whether or not they fulfil the inclusion criteria.

During data collection, it may be useful for reviewers to indicate the source page numbers against each item recorded; this facilitates later comparisons of extracted data.

Following completion of Sections 1 and 2, reviewers should reach agreement for each item on the checklist. If the study does not fulfil the study criteria, no further data should be extracted.

If the study fulfils the inclusion criteria, the reviewers should agree the study design, and fill in the appropriate version of Section 3 (RCT, CBA, ITS).

Discrepancies between reviewers completing Sections 1 and 2 should be resolved by discussion. *Decisions that cannot be resolved easily should be referred to the research fellow, for discussion by the panel.*

In all sections, data which are missing or not clear in a published report should be marked clearly on the data collection form. If time permits, missing information will be sought from the contact author of a paper by the research fellow.

Items which are clearly not applicable to the study in question should be marked accordingly.

Section 1: Inclusion criteria
Scope
The scope of the review is interventions to promote a healthy diet in women of childbearing age and women who are pregnant.

The target population is 'free-living' women and specifically excludes groups of women who are at clinically-defined high risk of diet-related disease, e.g. diabetic women, malnourished women. In general, where there is doubt about whether or not to include a study on these grounds, it should be included and attention drawn to the possible high risk issue.

All interventions aimed at improving diet should be included, irrespective of whether the investigators' explicit or implicit interest is in improving pregnancy or other health/disease outcomes.

Design
The review aims to include randomised controlled trials, controlled before and after studies and interrupted time series analyses. The basic criteria for including/excluding on this basis are incorporated into the table. For many studies, it may be difficult to assess every criterion with confidence, and a '?' should be entered if there is genuine uncertainty. Reviewers should work through the questions and attempt to answer them all before they try to decide on the study design. When making this decision, reviewers should assess first whether it fulfils the criteria for an RCT; second, for a CBA; third for an ITS. If there are still difficulties, the paper should be discussed and agreed between the two reviewers; if there is still uncertainty, it should be referred to the third reviewer for a final decision. All studies in this category should be put 'on hold' until a definite decision on its design has been agreed.

Relevance/interpretability
Every attempt should be made to find appropriate data and results, even if they are presented in a confusing format. Any papers which fulfil the scope and design criteria, but appear to fail the interpretability criteria, should be passed on to the third reviewer for final confirmation of its exclusion.

Section 2: Interventions

This section should be completed for all studies, whether or not they are to be included in the main review. State all interventions for each intervention and control group.

(*Note*: The categories are not mutually exclusive.)

Type of intervention
- education – altering knowledge
- counselling – giving advice
- technological – modification to environment
- policy – alteration of normal practice as agreed by a competent decision-making body
- other (specify, describe)

Target population
- pregnant women alone (all ages)
- pregnant women alone (teenagers specifically)
- non-pregnant women of childbearing age alone
- all women of childbearing age, pregnant or non-pregnant
- women of childbearing age as part of a larger population

Purpose of intervention
- improve pregnancy outcomes alone
- improve pregnancy outcomes and other outcomes
- improve other health outcomes

Aims of intervention
Describe the nature of desired change according to the authors, e.g.
- improved diet (specify)
- weight management
- other (specify)

Medium employed
individual contact
- health professional
- non-health professional
- volunteer
- peer
- other (specify)

no individual contact
- recorded media (video, audiotape)
- computer
- written material
- broadcast media
- other (specify)

Recipient	● individual
	● family
	● group – specify nature
	● community
	● 'influential third party' – i.e. individual(s) having important influence on diet of target population
	● other (specify)

| *Timing* | ● frequency/number of intervention events |
| | ● overall duration of intervention |

Setting	● health care setting
	● community
	● workplace
	● educational establishment
	● other (specify)

| *Nature of control intervention* | ● summarise details |

Funding for intervention	● governmental organisation
	● commercial organisation
	● health care organisation
	● voluntary/charitable body
	● other (specify)

Section 3

A. Quality of study design: randomised controlled trials

Unit of allocation (i.e. who or what was allocated to intervention and control groups)

Individual
Group
Community
Other (specify)
NOT CLEAR

Unit of analysis (e.g. results analysed as average change in outcome per person or per group)

Individual
Group
Community
Other (specify)
NOT CLEAR

Power calculation (i.e. whether the study has sufficient power to detect clinically important effects as statistically significant)

> PRESENT – if power calculations given (record the power)
> NOT CLEAR – if it is not clear whether a power calculation is reported
> ABSENT – if no power calculation stated

Concealment of allocation (i.e. protection against selection bias)

> YES if:
> (a)   any random process of allocation to intervention and control groups is described explicitly, e.g. the use of random number tables
> and
> (b)   there was some form of centralised randomisation scheme, an on-site computer system or sealed opaque envelopes were used
>
> NOT CLEAR if:
> (a)   the allocation procedure is not described explicitly but terms such as 'random' are used without further explanation
> and/or
> (b)   the authors report using a 'list' or 'table', 'envelopes' or 'sealed envelopes' for allocation
>
> NO if:
> (a)   the authors report using alternation such as reference to case record numbers, dates of birth, day of the week or any other such approach
> and/or
> (b)   the authors report using any allocation process that is entirely transparent before assignment, such as an open list of random numbers or assignments
> and/or
> (c)   allocation was altered (by investigators, professionals or patients/subjects)

Follow-up of study subjects (i.e. protection against exclusion bias)

> YES if outcome measures obtained for 80–100 per cent of subjects randomised; do not assume 100 per cent follow-up unless stated explicitly
> NOT CLEAR if not specified in the paper
> NO if outcome measures obtained for less than 80 per cent of subjects randomised

*Blinded assessment of primary outcome(s)** (i.e. protection against detection bias)

YES if:

(a) the authors state explicitly that the primary outcome variables were assessed blindly (without knowledge of whether the individual was in intervention or control group)

(b) the outcome variables are objective, e.g. biochemical measurements of nutrient levels in blood samples, responses to self-completion dietary questionnaire.

NOT CLEAR if not specified in the paper or unable to assess

NO if the outcomes were not assessed blindly, e.g. dietary habits assessed by interviewer who was aware of whether the subject was in intervention or control group

Baseline measurement

YES if outcomes were measured prior to the intervention, and no substantial differences were present across intervention and control groups

NOT CLEAR if baseline measures are not reported, or if it is unclear whether baseline measures are substantially different across study groups

NOT DONE if there are differences at baseline in main outcome measures likely to undermine the post-intervention differences (e.g. are differences between the groups before the intervention similar to those found post-intervention?)

Protection against contamination (i.e. behaviour in control group influenced by exposure in some way to the intervention)

YES if allocation was by community, institution or clinic and it is unlikely that the control group received the intervention

NOT CLEAR if subjects were allocated within a setting where it is possible that communication between intervention and control subjects could have occurred

NO if it is likely that the control group received the intervention (e.g. cross-over trial)

*Primary outcome(s) are those variables that correspond to the primary hypothesis or question as defined by the authors. In the event that some of the primary outcome variables were assessed in a blind fashion and others were not, score each separately and label each outcome variable clearly

Section 3
A. Quality of study design: controlled before and after studies

Unit of allocation (i.e. who or what was allocated to study groups)

> Individual
> Group
> Community
> Other (specify)
> NOT CLEAR

Unit of analysis (e.g. results analysed as average change in outcome per person or per group)

> Individual
> Group
> Community
> Other (specify)
> NOT CLEAR

Power calculation (i.e. whether the study has sufficient power to detect clinically important effects as statistically significant)

> PRESENT – if power calculations given (record the power)
> NOT CLEAR – if it is not clear whether a power calculation is reported
> ABSENT – if no power calculation stated

Baseline measurement

> YES if outcomes were measured prior to the intervention, and no substantial differences were present across study groups (e.g. where multiple pre-intervention measures describe similar trends in intervention and control groups)
> NOT CLEAR if baseline measures are not reported, or if it is unclear whether baseline measures are substantially different across study groups
> NO if there are differences at baseline in main outcome measures likely to undermine the post-intervention differences (e.g. are differences between the groups before the intervention similar to those found post-intervention?)

Blinded assessment of primary outcome(s) ★ (protection against detection bias)

> YES if:
> (a) the authors state explicitly that the primary outcome

★Primary outcome(s) are those variables that correspond to the primary hypothesis or question as defined by the authors. In the event that some of the primary outcome variables were assessed in a blind fashion and others were not, score each separately on the back of the form and label each outcome variable clearly

variables were assessed blindly (without knowledge of whether the individual was in intervention or control group)

(b) the outcome variables are objective, e.g. biochemical measurements of nutrient levels in blood samples, responses to self-completion dietary questionnaire

NOT CLEAR if not specified in the paper or unable to assess

NO if the outcomes were not assessed blindly, e.g. dietary habits assessed by interviewer who was aware of whether the subject was in intervention or control group

Protection against contamination (i.e. behaviour in control group influenced by exposure in some way to the intervention)

YES if allocation was by community, institution or clinic and it is unlikely that the control group received the intervention

NOT CLEAR if subjects were allocated within a setting where it is possible that communication between intervention and control subjects could have occurred

NO if it is likely that the control group received the intervention (e.g. cross-over trial)

Follow-up of study subjects (i.e. protection against exclusion bias)

YES if outcome measures obtained for 80–100 per cent of subjects randomised; do not assume 100 per cent follow-up unless stated explicitly

NOT CLEAR if not specified in the paper

NO if outcome measures obtained for less than 80 per cent of subjects randomised

Section 3
B. Details of participants (all studies)

Age   Give mean age of participants (state NOT CLEAR if information not available)

Country   State NOT CLEAR if information not available

Other characteristics (for each state NOT CLEAR if information not available)

(a) Ethnicity
(b) Socioeconomic group
(c) Other (specify)

The number included in each intervention or control group (i.e. the number of 'units' which entered each group in the study – will normally be individuals, but may be groups or communities): for each, state NOT CLEAR if information not available

Ethical approval

YES if ethical approval sought and obtained for the study
NOT CLEAR if not reported

Section 3
C. Nutrition outcomes (all studies)
Describe the type of nutrition outcome measures

Behavioural
Biochemical
Anthropometric
Other (specify)

Describe main nutrition outcome measure(s)
Report all the main outcomes described by the authors

Length of time during which outcomes were measured after initiation of the intervention

Length of time during which outcomes were measured after the intervention ended

Is there a post intervention follow-up period to examine deterioration?

YES
NOT CLEAR
NO

Briefly describe any non-nutrition outcome measures used, e.g. birth-weight, length of gestation, etc.

Section 3
D. Results: randomised controlled trials
Main results

State the main results of the nutrition outcome(s), for each study group, in natural units

Differences between groups post-intervention

For each available comparison, give the post-intervention differences between study groups, in natural units. Include statistical significance if reported for these differences, *only if* the units of allocation and analysis are the same.

In all cases, report a more favourable outcome in the intervention group as a positive (+) finding (i.e. where differences in the groups are in the intended direction).

Describe results for non-nutrition outcomes in similar format to nutrition outcomes, if possible

Section 3
D: Results: controlled before and after studies
Main results
State the main results of the main outcome(s), for each study group, in natural units

Pre- post-intervention differences in outcome(s)

For each study group, calculate the pre- post-intervention difference for each outcome in natural units (i.e. the post-intervention outcome minus the pre-intervention outcome).

Differences across intervention and control groups

For each available comparison, calculate the difference across study groups of the pre- post-intervention change (i.e. if, for an outcome measure, ΔE is the pre- post-intervention change in the intervention group, and ΔC is the pre- post-intervention change in the control group, this will be $\Delta E - \Delta C$).

Include statistical significance if reported for these differences, *only if* the units of allocation and analysis are the same.

In all cases, report a more favourable outcome in the intervention group as a positive (+) finding (i.e. where differences in the groups are in the intended direction).

Results as summarised for review

State the results as they will be entered in the review, and describe how calculated (e.g. relative percentage differences attributable to the intervention).

Describe results for non-nutrition outcomes in similar format to nutrition outcomes, if possible.

Section 1: Inclusion criteria

Aspects of the study	Insert ✓ X ?	Criteria
1. Did the study include women of childbearing age (pregnant or non-pregnant)?		Scope
2. Was an intervention described which aimed to improve diet?		Scope
3. Were baseline data collected before the intervention?		RCT CBA ITS
4. If (3) yes, were baseline data collected for at least two points in time?		ITS
5. Did the intervention occur at a clearly defined point in time?		RCT CBA ITS
6. Were outcome data collected after the intervention?		RCT CBA ITS
7. If (6) yes, were outcome data collected for at least two points in time?		ITS
8. Was there a control group?		RCT CBA
9. If (8) yes, was the control group concurrent?		RCT CBA
10. If (8) yes, were subjects allocated to groups on any kind of random or pseudo-random basis?		RCT
11. If (10) no, were intervention and control groups comparable for main risk/confounding variables?		CBA
12. If (10) no, were data collected from intervention and control groups contemporaneously?		CBA
13. Are relevant and interpretable data presented?		R/I

A. SCOPE criteria
Both scope criteria must be met – if yes, assess DESIGN criteria

B. DESIGN criteria
Eligible if   all RCT criteria ticked (irrespective of other criteria)
               or
               all CBA criteria ticked (irrespective of other criteria)
               or
               all ITS criteria ticked (irrespective of other criteria)

If meets the criteria for RCT, CBA or ITS – assess RELEVANCE/INTERPRETABILITY criteria

C. RELEVANCE/INTERPRETABILITY criteria
Eligible if R/I box ticked

If A, B and C satisfied then the study should be included in the main review.

Section 2: Interventions

Type of intervention

Target population

Purpose of intervention

Aims
(nutrition)

Aims
(non-nutrition, e.g. pregnancy outcomes)

Medium employed

Recipient

Timing

Setting

Nature of control intervention

Funding for intervention

Section 3
A. Quality of study design: randomised controlled trials

Unit of allocation

Unit of analysis

Power calculation

Concealment of allocation

Follow-up of study subjects

Blinded assessment of primary outcome(s)

Baseline measurement

Protection against contamination

Section 3
B. Details of participants

Mean age of participants

Country

Ethnicity

Socioeconomic group

Other characteristics

Number in intervention group

Number in control group (1)

Number in control group (2)*

Ethical approval

*If more than two control groups, please give further details overleaf

Section 3
C. Outcomes

**Types of outcome measures
(nutrition)**

Details of outcome measures

**Length of time during which outcomes were
measured after initiation of the intervention**

**Length of time during which outcomes were
measured after the intervention ended**

**Is there a post-intervention follow-up period
to examine deterioration?**

**Types of outcome measures
(non-nutrition)**

Section 3
D. Results

Result	Differences between groups post-intervention	Statistical significance	Results summarised for review
NUTRITION			
NON-NUTRITION			

Section 3
A. Quality of study design: controlled before and after studies

Unit of allocation

Unit of analysis

Power calculation

Follow-up of study subjects

Blinded assessment of primary outcome(s)

Baseline measurement

Protection against contamination

Section 3

B. Details of participants

Mean age of participants

Country

Ethnicity

Socioeconomic group

Other characteristics

Number in intervention group

Number in control group (1)

Number in control group (2)*

Ethical approval

*If more than two control groups please give further details overleaf

Section 3
C. Outcomes

**Types of outcome measures
(nutrition)**

Details of outcome measures

**Length of time during which outcomes were
measured after initiation of the intervention**

**Length of time during which outcomes were
measured after the intervention ended**

**Is there a post-intervention follow-up period
to examine deterioration?**

**Types of outcome measures
(non-nutrition)**

Section 3
D. Results

Result	Pre- post-intervention difference for intervention on group ΔE	Pre- post-intervention difference for control group(s) ΔC	Pre- post-intervention across groups $\Delta E-\Delta C$	Statistical significance	Results summarised for review
NUTRITION					
NON-NUTRITION					

Appendix D. Commentary on the WIC Program

The special supplemental food programme for women, infants and children (WIC Program) has been funded by the US Department of Agriculture since 1972 and is intended to provide food supplements for low income pregnant and post-partum women and children under 5 years of age who are considered to be at nutritional risk. The purpose of the WIC Program for pregnant women is to improve pregnancy outcomes, including rates of prematurity and infant and foetal mortality. The programme is administered at state level, delivered by a wide variety of agencies, and gives priority to geographical areas with high rates of infant mortality, low birthweight and low income. The number of potentially eligible participants exceeds the funds available so each state is forced to form criteria for allocating the benefits.

The elements of the WIC Program are: 1. supplemental food tailored to individual needs, usually in the form of a monthly allotment of milk, cheese, eggs and other nutrient dense foods, generally targeting intakes of protein, iron, calcium, vitamin A and vitamin C; 2. a minimum of two sessions of nutrition education for enrolled individuals every six months, with the format at the discretion of the provider; and 3. assistance in gaining access to health care services (although the programme itself does not pay for health services).

Although published evaluations of the WIC Program generally fell outside the scope of this review, we considered it would be useful to provide a commentary on the current evidence of its effectiveness. It should be noted, however, that our search strategy was not designed to capture all WIC evaluations in a systematic and comprehensive manner, although we believe we have identified the key publications from 1985 to the time of conducting this review.

A total of twelve published articles on WIC within the time frame of our review were identified (Metcoff *et al.*, 1985; Schramm, 1985, 1986; Stockbauer, 1986, 1987; Rush *et al.*, 1988a–e; Buescher *et al.*, 1993; Brown, Watkins and Hiett, 1996). These included reviews and commentaries (Rush *et al.*, 1988b, 1988d); as well as reports of evaluation studies (Metcoff *et al.*, 1985; Schramm, 1985, 1986; Stockbauer, 1986, 1987; Rush *et al.*, 1988a, 1988c, 1988e; Buescher *et al.*, 1993; Brown, Watkins and Hiett, 1996) conducted usually at the behest of the US Congress and the various state authorities. These evaluations in the main take the form of: 1. retrospective analyses linking administrative data on WIC participation with routinely available outcome data (for example data from birth certificates, Medicaid records, etc.) or 2. controlled before-and-after studies in which outcomes in WIC participants are compared with outcomes in non-randomly selected groups of non-WIC participants. Such studies are inevitably subject to the positive bias inherent in non-randomised designs. We were able to identify only one randomised controlled trial (Metcoff et al., 1985) published in our time frame of interest.

The primary outcomes reported in these evaluations are usually birthweight and related variables, and standard statistical techniques are used to adjust for potential confounding biological, clinical and socio-demographic factors. Only three of the studies (Metcoff et al., 1985; Rush et al., 1988c, 1988e; Brown, Watkins and Hiett, 1996) (Rush and colleagues reporting results over two papers) evaluated maternal nutrition outcomes separately. These all tend to support a beneficial effect of WIC participation, but are all confounded to a certain extent by baseline differences between the WIC and non-WIC comparison groups. Of these only one (Rush et al., 1988c, 1988e) presents an analysis relating the separate effects on maternal nutrition of the food supplements and the nutrition education components of the WIC Program; in this case this assessment is based on the response to a single, unvalidated question, in a follow-up survey.

Given the methodological difficulties noted above, the overall conclusion is that there is equivocal evidence for the effectiveness of the WIC Program in producing positive effects on birthweight and other factors which influence infant mortality. Food supplementation for pregnant women at high risk because of low income, deleterious health behaviours such as smoking, or a past history of delivering a low birthweight infant may produce benefits in terms of higher mean birthweights and lower proportion of low birthweight infants. However, the effect of supplementation in other pregnant women remains questionable. It is impossible to draw conclusions regarding the independent effect of the nutrition education component over and above the supplementation element.

We would tend to agree with the conclusion of Rush and colleagues after reviewing the evidence from the National WIC Evaluation project: 'after a decade of the existence of the program, there existed too little information to judge, one way or the other, whether WIC was meeting the goals set for it by the Congress and the public'. (Rush et al., 1988d).

Appendix E. Search strategy

The electronic searching took place in two phases. In the first phase, a search for reviews and meta-analyses was conducted. This was followed by a search for original source material. The following Ovid MEDLINE search strategies formed the basis of searches on the other databases also. They were based on CRD guidelines (NHS Centre for Reviews and Dissemination 1996).

Phase 1: Systematic reviews and meta-analyses
Part one: Design terms
1   (meta-analysis or review literature).sh.
2   meta-analy$ or (meta adj anal$).tw.
3   metaanal$.tw.
4   meta-analysis.pt.
5   review, academic.pt.
6   review literature.pt.
7   case report.sh.
8   letter.pt.
9   historical article.pt.
10 review of reported cases.pt.
11 review, multicase.pt.
12 or/1–6
13 or/7–11
14 12 not 13
15 animal.sh.
16 human.sh.
17 15 not (15 and 16)
18 14 not 17

Part two: Specific subject terms
19 exp health behavior/
20 exp life style/
21 exp health promotion/
22 exp health education/
23 wellness program$.tw.
24 exp community health services/
25 exp preventive health services/
26 exp preventive medicine/
27 exp community health centers/
28 health behavior.tw
29 life style.tw
30 health promotion.tw
31 health education.tw
32 preventive health services.tw
33 preventive medicine.tw
34 community health centers.tw

35 community health services.tw
36 health behavi$r.tw
37 health$ adj15 campaign$.tw.
38 behavior$ adj15 modifi$.tw.
39 or/19–38

Part three: Content/topic terms
40 (health$ adj5 eat$).ti,ab,sh.
41 ((evaluat$ adj15 health promotion) or health education).ti,ab,sh.
42 exp food/
43 exp diet/
44 exp nutrition/
45 healthy eating.tw.
46 food.tw
47 diet.tw
48 nutrition.tw
49 exp nutrition/ed
50 fruit$.ti,ab,sh. or vegetable$.tw.
51 low$ adj25 Fat$
52 exp food habits/
53 food habits.tw
54 ((adhere$ or efficacy or maintain$) adj15 diet).ti,ab,sh.
55 or/40–54
56 18 and 39
57 55 and 56

Phase 2: Primary sources (reports of studies)
Part one: Research design terms
1   randomized controlled trial.pt.
2   controlled clinical trial.pt.
3   randomized controlled trials.sh.
4   random allocation.sh.
5   double blind method.sh.
6   single blind method.sh.
7   clinical trial.pt.
8   exp clinical trials/
9   (clin$ adj25 trial$).tw.
10 ((singl$ or doubl$ or trebl$ or tripl$) adj25 (blind$ or mask$)).tw.
11 placebos.sh.
12 placebo$.tw.
13 random$.tw.
14 (clin$ and trial$).ti.
15 (clin$ and trial$).ab.
16 (control$ and trial$).ti.
17 (control$ and trial$).ab.
18 (experimental adj15 design).tw.
19 research design.sh.

20 experimental design.tw.
21 exp intervention studies/
22 exp evaluation studies/
23 exp program evaluation/
24 or/1–23

Part two: Health promotion theory/topic terms
25 exp health behavior/
26 exp life style/
27 exp health promotion/
28 exp health education/
29 wellness program$.tw.
30 exp community health services/
31 exp preventive health services/
32 exp preventive medicine/
33 exp community health centers/
34 health behavi$r.tw
35 life style.tw
36 health promotion.tw
37 health education.tw
38 community health services.tw
39 preventive health services.tw
40 preventive medicine.tw
41 community health centers.tw
42 health$ adj15 campaign$.tw.
43 behavior$ adj15 modifi$.tw.
44 or/25–43
45 24 and 44

Part three: Healthy eating/diet/nutrition content terms
46 (health$ adj5 eat$).ti,ab,sh.
47 evaluat$ adj15 health promotion) or health education).ti,ab,sh.
48 exp food/
49 exp diet/
50 exp nutrition/
51 exp nutrition/ed
52 fruit$.ti,ab,sh. or vegetable$.tw.
53 low$ adj25 fat$
54 exp food habits/
55 exp food habits/px
56 food habits.tw
57 food.tw
58 diet.tw
59 nutrition.tw
60 healthy eating.tw
61 ((adhere$ or efficacy or maintain$) adj15 diet).ti,ab,sh.
62 or/46–61
63 45 and 62

Appendix F. Details of study designs

Study characteristics – women of childbearing age

Study	Participants and setting	Intervention and duration	Methods	Control group/ intervention	Outcomes
Johnson, Howell, and Molloy (1993) Ireland RCT	Age range: mean 23.6 SE background: ≥ 87% manual classes; first-time mothers Setting: Community Intervention = 141 Control = 121	Aim: to improve infant development Education Counselling Monthly 1 year	Unit of allocation: Individual Unit of analysis: Individual Power calculation: No Concealment of allocation: Unclear Follow-up > 80%: Yes Blinded assessment of primary outcome: Unclear Baseline equivalence: Unclear Reliable outcome measure: Unclear Protection against contamination: Unclear	Standard public health nurse support	'Appropriate' or 'inappropriate' intake levels of indicators (animal and non-animal protein, wholefoods, vegetables, fruit, milk, energy) for mothers and infants Assessed at child's first birthday
Fine et al. (1994) UK RCT	Age range: 25–34 SE background: socioeconomic groups C2, D, E Setting: Community Intervention 1 = 87 Intervention 2 = 86 Control = 91	Aim: improve diet as per COMA recommendations Education (two levels) One-off	Unit of allocation: Individual Unit of analysis: Individual* Power calculation: No Concealment of allocation: Unclear Follow-up > 80%: Unclear Blinded assessment of primary outcome: Unclear Baseline equivalence: Unclear Reliable outcome measure: Unclear Protection against contamination: Unclear *Not analysed strictly by intention to treat	Data collection only	Score in a nutrition knowledge questionnaire 1 week after intervention
Brown, Lee and Oyomopito (1996) Australia CBA	Age range: 32–65 SE background: Greek extraction. Setting: Community Intervention = 26 Control = 22	Aim: promote heart health through reducing fat intake and promoting exercise Education Exercise programme Weekly 12 weeks	Unit of allocation: Group Unit of analysis: Individual Power calculation: No Follow-up > 80%: Yes Blinded assessment of primary outcome: Unclear Baseline equivalence: Yes Reliable outcome measure: Yes Protection against contamination: Yes	Neighbourhood control group, data collection only Offered deferred intervention	Self-report nutrition behaviour Anthropometric and fitness measurements End of intervention and 12 weeks later

Study characteristics – women of childbearing age (contd)

Study	Participants and setting	Intervention and duration	Methods	Control group/ intervention	Outcomes
Cox et al. (1995) USA CBA or RCT?	Age range: 20–45 SE background: low income, some pregnant Setting: Community Intervention 1 = 113 Intervention 2 = 116 Control = 110	*Aim:* improve cancer risk by improving diet Education (two levels) Over 6 months	Unit of allocation: Individual Unit of analysis: Individual Power calculation: No Concealment of allocation: Unclear Follow-up > 80%: Unclear . Blinded assessment of primary outcome: Unclear Baseline equivalence: Unclear Reliable outcome measure: Unclear Protection against contamination: Unclear	Money management lessons	Self-report nutrition behaviour At end of 6-month intervention period
Tucker, Harris and Martin (1996) USA RCT	Age range: 23–66 SE background: 40% college education Setting: Community Intervention = 30+ Control = 30+	*Aim:* improve usual diet through strength training Strength training Usual diet 12 weeks	Unit of allocation: Individual Unit of analysis: Individual Power calculation: Yes Concealment of allocation: Unclear Follow-up > 80%: Yes Blinded assessment of primary outcome: Yes Baseline equivalence: Yes Reliable outcome measure: Yes Protection against contamination: Unclear	Flexibility training for 12 weeks while consuming usual diet	Self-report nutrition behaviour Anthropometric measurements At baseline, 6 and 12 weeks

Study characteristics – women who are pregnant

Study	Participants and setting	Intervention and duration	Methods	Control group/ intervention	Outcomes
Anderson, Campbell and Shepherd (1995) UK RCT	Age range: mean 26 SE background: 30% non-manual (RG) Setting: Clinic Intervention = 111 Control = 145	*Aim*: test nutrition knowledge, attitudes and behaviour following intervention Education 2 mailshots, one at booking and one at 26 weeks	Unit of allocation: Individual Unit of analysis: Individual Power calculation: No Concealment of allocation: No Follow-up > 80%: Yes Blinded assessment of primary outcome: Yes Baseline equivalence: Yes Reliable outcome measure: Yes Protection against contamination: Unclear	Usual care (includes general health education)	Nutrition knowledge Nutrition attitude Self-report nutrition behaviour At 30 weeks' gestation
Kafatos, Vlachonikolis and Codrington (1989) Greece RCT	Age range: mean 23 SE background: >70% Low SES Setting: Community Intervention = 300 Control = 268	*Aim*: improve maternal diet and weight gain in pregnancy Education Counselling Enrolment to term	Unit of allocation: Clinic Unit of analysis: Individual Power calculation: No Concealment of allocation: Yes Follow-up > 80%: Unclear Blinded assessment of primary outcome: No Baseline equivalence: Unclear Reliable outcome measure: Yes Protection against contamination: Yes	? Data collection only	Self-report nutrition behaviour Nutrition biomarkers Weight gain during pregnancy Every 4 weeks from 21 weeks' gestation until term
Sweeney et al. (1985) US RCT	Age range: mean 23.1 SE background: some WIC enrollees Setting: Clinic Intervention = 22 Control = 21	*Aim*: improve diet/ weight gain in pregnancy Diet prescription Education plus video 20 weeks	Unit of allocation: Individual Unit of analysis: Individual Power calculation: No Concealment of allocation: Unclear Follow-up > 80%: Yes Blinded assessment of primary outcome: No Baseline equivalence: Yes Reliable outcome measure: Unclear Protection against contamination: Unclear	Prescription not communicated plus control video	Self-report consumption of prescription Self-report nutrition behaviour Weight gain during pregnancy Every 2–4 weeks from 20 weeks' gestation until term

Study characteristics – women who are pregnant (contd)

Study	Participants and setting	Intervention and duration	Methods	Control group/intervention	Outcomes
Villar et al. (1992)/ Belizán et al. (1995) Argentina, Brazil, Cuba, Mexico RCT	Age range: mean 24.4 SE background: High-risk LBW Setting: Community Intervention = 1115 Control = 1120	*Aim:* increase social support and health education Education Counselling 4–6 home visits through pregnancy	Unit of allocation: Individual Unit of analysis: Individual Power calculation: Yes Concealment of allocation: Yes Follow-up > 80%: Yes Blinded assessment of primary outcome: Yes Baseline equivalence: Yes Reliable outcome measure: Unclear Protection against contamination: Unclear	Routine prenatal care	Self-report nutrition behaviour Self-report consumption of supplements At 36 weeks gestation. Plus obstetric outcomes

Appendix G. Detailed results tables

Selected detailed results – women of childbearing age

Study	Main outcome measure	Allocation	Main effect		Absolute before–after difference	% change over baseline	Absolute between-group difference[a]	Comments
			Before	After	After–Before[a]	Rounded to nearest %[a]		
Brown, Lee and Oyomopito (1996) Australia	Fat habit scores		Mean (SD) [N]	Mean (SD) [N]				
CBA		Con	4.00 (1.52) [20]	3.75 (2.00) [17]	−0.25	−6	−1.55	
		Exp	3.15 (1.74) [26]	2.20 (1.47) [25]	−0.95	−30		
	Total cholesterol (mmol/l)	Con	5.36 (0.71) [20]	5.47 (0.77) [17]	(+0.11)	(+2)	(+0.28)	
		Exp	5.65 (1.19) [26]	5.75 (0.84) [24]	(+0.1)	(+2)		
	Triglycerides (mmol/l)	Con	1.25 (0.51) [19]	1.27 (0.50) [17]	(+0.02)	(+1)	(+0.44)	
		Exp	1.60 (1.38) [24]	1.71 (2.58) [24]	(+0.21)	(+13)		
	Body mass index (kg/m²)	Con	28.9 (4.5) [22]	28.8 (4.3) [21]	−0.1	<1	−0.7	
		Exp	29.8 (5.5) [26]	28.1 (4.8) [25]	−1.7	−6		
	Estimated fat (%) at baseline, end of intervention	Con	41.7 (4.5) [22]	41.3 (4.4) [21]	−0.4	−1	−0.6	
		Exp	41.8 (4.1) [26]	40.7 (4.4) [25]	−1.1	−3		
Cox et al. (1995) USA	Self-reported intake (24-h recall) of:		Data not reported	Data not reported	Reported mean (SE) change		Difference in changes	
CBA/RCT	energy (kcal)	Con[b]			(+171 (56))		(+56)	
		Exp 1[b]			(+227 (52))		−68	
		Exp 2[b]			(+103 (60))			
	fat (% energy)	Con			−0.3 (0.8)			
		Exp 1			−3.7 (0.7)		−3.4	
		Exp 2			−4.9 (0.8)		−4.6	
	dietary fibre (g)	Con			+2.2 (0.9)			
		Exp 1			+3.7 (0.6)		+1.5	
	at baseline, end of intervention	Exp 2			+5.5 (0.7)		+3.3	

[a]Parentheses indicate change opposite to desired direction [b]Con = control; Exp1 = Group E; Exp 2 = Group EC; in report

Selected detailed results – women of childbearing age (contd)

Study	Main outcome measure	Allocation	Main effect		Absolute before–after difference	% change over baseline	Absolute between-group difference[a]	Comments
			Before	After	After–Before[a]	Rounded to nearest %[a]		
Fine *et al* (1994) UK	Knowledge score (maximum = 36)	Con[b]	Mean[c] [N] 14.3 [91]	Mean[c] [N] 16.8 [91]	+2.5	+17		Not possible to assess statistical significance as standard deviations not reported.
		Exp 1[b]	14.7 [87]	20.2 [87]	+5.5	+37	+3.4	
RCT		Exp 2[b]	16.6 [86]	21.3 [86]	+4.7	+28	+4.5	
	at baseline, one week after intervention							
Johnson, Howell and Molloy (1993) Ireland	Self-reported intake (24-h recall) of		Data not reported	Percentage 'appropriate' [total N]	Not estimable	Not estimable	Percentage points	
RCT	wholefoods	Con		24 [105]				
		Exp		84 [127]			60[d]	
	vegetables	Con		43 [105]				
		Exp		81 [127]			38[d]	
	fruit	Con		28 [105]				
		Exp		55 [127]			27[d]	
	total energy	Con		53 [105]				
	at end of intervention	Exp		94 [127]			41[d]	

[a]Parentheses indicate change opposite to desired direction [b]Con = 'baseline'; Exp 1 = 'control'; Exp 2 = 'test' in report [c]Reconstructed from reported data [d]*p* < 0.05

Selected detailed results – women of childbearing age (contd)

Study	Main outcome measure	Allocation	Main effect			Absolute before–after difference	% change over baseline	Absolute between-group differenceª	Comments
				Before	After	After–Beforeª	Rounded to nearest %ª		
			Mean (SD) [N]	Mean (SD) [N]	Mean (SD) [N]				
Tucker, Harris and Martin (1996) USA	Self- reported intakes (7d record) of:								
	energy (kcal)	Con		1 996 (402) [30]	1 911 (431) [30]	−85	−4		
		Exp		2 004 (427) [30]	1 779 (398) [30]	−225	−11	−132	
RCT	fat ('% diet')	Con		32.1 (5.7) [30]	33.1 (4.7) [30]	(+1)	(+3)		
		Exp		34.2 (5.1) [30]	29.7 (4.1) [30]	−4.5	−13	−3.4	
	carbohydrate ('% diet')	Con		53.0 (6.4) [30]	52.3 (4.7) [30]	(−0.7)	(−1)		
		Exp		51.4 (6.2) [30]	55.6 (5.3) [30]	+4.2	+8	+3.3	
	protein ('% diet')	Con		14.9 (3.7) [30]	14.6 (2.0) [30]	−0.3	−2		
		Exp		14.4 (2.3) [30]	14.7 (2.8) [30]	(+0.3)	(+2)	+0.1	
	at baseline, 12 weeks								

ªParentheses indicate change opposite to desired direction

Selected detailed results – women who are pregnant

Study	Main outcome measure	Allocation	Main effect		Absolute before–after difference After–Before[a]	% change over baseline Rounded to nearest %[a]	Absolute between-group difference[a]	Comments
			Before	After Mean (SD) [N]				
Anderson, Campbell and Shepherd (1995) UK	Nutrition knowledge scores		Data not reported		Not estimable	Not estimable		
RCT	nutrition terms (max = 3)	Con Exp		1.4 (1.1) [146] 1.4 (1.0) [142]			0	
	theoretical principles (max = 5)	Con Exp		2.7 (1.2) [146] 2.9 (1.3) [142]			+0.2	
	practical application (max = 11)	Con Exp		5.9 (1.9) [145] 6.7 (1.9) [141]			+0.8	
	total score (max = 19)	Con Exp		10.0 (3.2) [145] 10.9 (3.4) [141]			+0.9	
	Attitude scores (range of possibles) behavioural intention (–3 to +3)	Con Exp		1.7 (1.4) [146] 1.8 (1.2) [142]			+0.1	
	direct attitudes (–12 to +12)	Con Exp		7.5 (3.8) [146] 7.6 (3.9) [142]			+0.1	
	direct subjective norm (–6 to +6)	Con Exp		0.4 (3.1) [146] 0.6 (3.2) [142]			+0.2	
	estimated attitude (–54 to +54)	Con Exp		17.7 (13.0) [146] 19.4 (12.8) [142]			+1.7	
	estimated subjective norm (–72 to +72)	Con Exp		9.1 (16.8) [146] 10.8 (19.1) [142]			+1.7	

[a]Parentheses indicate change opposite to desired direction

Selected detailed results – women who are pregnant (contd)

Study	Main outcome measure	Allocation	Main effect		Absolute before–after difference[a]	% change over baseline	Absolute between-group difference[a]	Comments
			Before	After	After–Before[a]	Rounded to nearest %[a]		
Anderson et al. (1995) (contd)	Self-reported intakes of		Data not reported	Mean (SD) [N]	Not estimable	Not estimable		
	energy (kJ)	Con		9489 (1843) [113]			−84	
		Exp		9405 (1986) [111]				
	fat (% energy)	Con		38.9 (4.9)			−0.8	
		Exp		38.1 (4.7)				
	carbohydrate (% energy)	Con		46.4 (4.8)			+0.3	
		Exp		46.7 (4.4)				
	fibre (g)	Con		20.2 (6.9)			+0.9	
		Exp		21.1 (7.1)				
	Proportion 'reaching dietary goal'							
	fat	Con		21 [113]				
		Exp		29 [111]				
	carbohydrate	Con		25 [113]				
		Exp		24 [111]				
	fibre	Con		39 [113]				
		Exp		39 [111]				
	at baseline, 30 weeks' gestation							

[a]Parentheses indicate change opposite to desired direction

Selected detailed results – women who are pregnant (contd)

Study	Main outcome measure	Allocation	Main effect Before	Main effect After	Absolute before-after difference After–Before[a]	% change over baseline Rounded to nearest %[a]	Absolute between-group difference[a]	Comments
Kafatos, Vlachonikolis and Codrington (1989) Greece RCT	Self-reported (24-h recall) and weighed intakes of energy (kcal)	Con Exp	Data not reported	Mean [N] 1685–1908 [180] 2103–2132 [216]	Not estimable	Not estimable	Not estimable	Not possible to quantify fat or carbohydrate intakes – presented as graphical data. Differences between groups apparently statistically significant but apparent baseline differences in carbohydrate intake.
	protein (g)	Con Exp		Median 63–69.5 [180] 72–76.7 [216]				
	at baseline, throughout pregnancy							
Sweeney et al. (1985) US RCT	Average daily prescription ingestion		Not applicable	Mean (SD) [N]	Not applicable	Not applicable		Aim of intervention was to promote protein and energy intake to improve obstetric outcomes.
	protein (g)	Con Exp		80.8 (21.9) [25] 91.6 (8.3) [18]			+10.8	
	protein (% prescription)	Con Exp		83.4 (35.0) [25] 88.9 (23.3) [18]			+5.5	
	energy (kcal)	Con Exp		2373 (538) [25] 2562 (423) [18]			+189	
	energy (% prescription)	Con Exp		81.9 (21.3) [25] 86.9 (15.3) [18]			+5	
	at baseline, through pregnancy							
Villar et al. (1992) Belizán et al. (1995) Argentina, Brazil, Cuba, Mexico RCT	Proportion reporting 'improvement in diet' as assessed by interview and dietitian	Con Exp	Percent [N] 58.5 [1120] 55.9 [1110]	Percent [N] 67.4 [1019] 67.7 [1009]	+8.9 +11.8	+15 +21	+0.3	
	at baseline, 36 weeks' gestation							

[a] Parentheses indicate change opposite to desired direction

Appendix H. Studies not included in review

Intervention studies
Subjects not free-living
Keim et al. (1996)

Wrong target group
Simkin-Silverman, Wing and Hansen (1995) – women approaching the menopause (age > 45)
Nunn, Newton and Foucher (1992) – men and women
Galletly et al. (1996) – infertile, obese women

Intervention not relevant
Kumanyika and Charleston (1992)
Bertram, Ventner and Stewart (1990)
Brodie and Slade (1990)
Cousins et al. (1992)
Czeizel and Dudas (1992)
Czeizel (1992)
Shah et al. (1996)
Agras et al. (1996)
Kennett and Ackerman (1995)

Non-random allocation and no/non-concurrent controls and/or no baseline data
Pregnancy:
Bruce and Tchabo (1989)
Perkin (1983)
Dubois et al. (1991)
Orstead et al. (1985)
Dow Allen and Ries (1985)
Taren and Graven (1991)
Metson et al. (1996)

Women of childbearing age:
Bower et al. (1996)
Quinn and Jenkins (1991)
Larsson and Lissner (1996)

No interpretable nutrition outcome data
All pregnancy:
McEnery and Rao (1986)
Heins et al. (1990)
Doyle et al. (1992)
Herman et al. (1996)

Duplicate reports
Kafatos *et al.* (1991)

Non-intervention studies identified by search strategy with appropriate target group
Pregnant women:
Anderson, Campbell and Shepherd (1993)
Anderson and Shepherd (1989)
Arkin (1986)
Bennett and McIlwaine (1985a)
Bennett and McIlwaine (1985b)
Brown, Buzzard, Jacobs Jr *et al.* (1996)
Schofield, Wheeler and Stewart (1988)
Loris, Dewey and Poirier-Brook (1985)
Lia-Hoagberg, Rode and Skovholt (1990)

Women of childbearing age:
Bjorkelund and Bengtsson (1994)
Devine and Sandstrom (1996)
Devine and Olson (1992)
Kennett and Ackerman (1995)
Megel *et al.* (1994)
Portsmouth *et al.* (1994)
Powell *et al.* (1994)
Reinli *et al.* (1996)
Sutherland *et al.* (1993)
Lissner *et al.* (1996)
McCargar *et al.* (1993)

References

Agras, W S, Berkowitz, R I, Arnow, B A, Telch, C F, Marnell, M, Henderson, J, Morris, Y and Wilfey, D E (1996). Maintenance following a very-low-calorie-diet. *Journal of Consulting and Clinical Psychology* **64**:610–13.

Anderson, A (1996). Eating for life. *Nursing Times* **90**:44–8.

Anderson, A S, Campbell, D M and Shepherd, R (1993). Nutrition knowledge, attitude to healthier eating and dietary intake in pregnant compared to non-pregnant women. *Journal of Human Nutrition and Dietetics* **6**:335–53.

Anderson, A S, Campbell, D M and Shepherd, R (1995). The influence of dietary advice on nutrient intake during pregnancy. *British Journal of Nutrition* **73**:163–77.

Anderson, A S and Shepherd, R (1989). Beliefs and attitudes toward 'healthier eating' among women attending maternity hospital. *Journal of Nutrition Education* **21**:208–12.

Andrien, M (1994). *Nutrition: a review of the effectiveness of health education and health promotion.* Utrecht: Dutch Centre for Health Promotion and Health Education.

Ajzen, I and Fishbein, M (1980). *Understanding attitudes and predicting social behaviour.* Englewood Cliffs, New Jersey: Prentice-Hall.

Arkin, E B (1986). Healthy mothers, healthy babies coalition: four years of progress. *Public Health Reports* **101**:147–56.

Barker, D J P (1992). *Fetal and infant origins of adult disease.* London: BMJ Publishing.

Barker, D J P (1998). The importance of early nutrition for long term health. *Nutrition Reviews* (in press).

Barker, D J P (ed.) (1994). *Mothers, babies and disease in later life.* London: BMJ Publishing.

Barker, W (1984). *The child development programme: a collaborative programme linking parents, community and health visitors.* Bristol: Early Childhood Development Unit, University of Bristol.

Baumslag, I N, Edelstein, T and Metz, J (1970). Reduction in incidence of prematurity by folic acid supplementation in pregnancy. *British Medical Journal* **260**:16–17.

Belizán, J M, Barros, F, Langer, A, Farnot, U, Victora, C and Villar, J (1995). Impact of health education during pregnancy on behavior and utilization of health resources. *American Journal of Obstetrics and Gynecology* **173**:894–9.

Bendich, A and Keen, C L (1993). Influence of maternal nutrition on pregnancy outcome. *Annals of New York Academy of Sciences* **678**:373–8.

Bennett, C A and McIlwaine, G (1985a). Health awareness and practices of primigravidae in Glasgow. *Health Bulletin* **43**:228–32.

Bennett, C A and McIlwaine, G (1985b). Study of antenatal vitamin and iron supplementation in Glasgow. *Health Bulletin* **43**:182–6.

Bero, L, Freemantle, N, Grilli, R *et al.* (eds) (1996a). *The Cochrane Collaboration on Effective Professional Practice: module of the Cochrane Database of Systematic Reviews.* 3rd edn. London: BMJ Publishing.

Bero, L, Freemantle, N, Grilli, R, Grimshaw, J M, Harvey, E and Oxman, A D (1996b). *Checklist for data abstraction in CCEPP reviews*. York: CCEPP (mimeo).

Bero, L, Grilli, R, Grimshaw, J and Oxman, A (eds) (1998). *The Cochrane Collaboration on Effective Professional Practice (CCEPP): Module of the Cochrane Database of Systematic Reviews*. The Cochrane Library, Issue 1 1998. Oxford: Update Software.

Bertram, S R, Venter, I and Stewart, R I (1990). Weight loss in obese women – exercise vs. dietary education. *South African Medical Journal* **78**:15–18.

Bjorkelund, C and Bengtsson, C (1994). Changing lifestyle: who benefits and how? Prevention in primary health care within the female population in a Swedish community. *Behaviour Change* **11**:145–52.

Block, G (1992). Fruit, vegetables and cancer prevention; a review of epidemiological evidence. *Nutrition & Cancer* **18**:1–29.

Bower, C, Blum, L, Watson, C and Stanley, F (1996). Folate and the prevention of neural tube defects: evaluation of a health promotion project in Western Australia. *Health Promotion International* **11**:177–87.

Bowman, M A and Spangler, J G (1995). Screening, health promotion, and prevention in women. *Primary Care* **22**:661–7.

Boyd, N R and Windsor, R A (1993). A meta-evaluation of nutrition education intervention research among pregnant women. *Health Education Quarterly* **20**:327–45.

Brodie, D A and Slade, P D (1990). Dietary versus healthy life style interventions in the treatment of obesity: resultant changes and the prediction of outcome. *Psychology and Health* **4**:319–31.

Brown, H L, Watkins, K and Hiett, A K (1996). The impact of Women, Infants and Children Food Supplement Program on birth outcome. *American Journal of Obstetrics and Gynecology* **174**:1279–83.

Brown, J E, Buzzard, I M, Jacobs, D R, Jr, Hannan, P J, Kushi, L H, Barosso, G M and Schmid, L A (1996). A food frequency questionnaire can detect pregnancy-related changes in diet. *American Dietetic Association Journal* **96**:262–6.

Brown, W J, Lee, C and Oyomopito, R (1996). Effectiveness of a bilingual heart health program for Greek-Australian women. *Health Promotion International* **11**:117–25.

Bruce, L and Tchabo, J G (1989). Nutrition intervention program in a prenatal clinic. *Obstetrics and Gynecology* **74**:310–12.

Buck, C and Donner, A (1982). The design of controlled experiments in the evaluation on non-therapeutic interventions. *Journal of Chronic Diseases* **35**:531–8.

Buescher, P A, Larson, L C, Nelson, M D, Jr and Lenihan, A J (1993). Prenatal WIC participation can reduce low birthweight and newborn medical costs: a cost-benefit analysis of WIC participation in North Carolina. *American Dietetic Association Journal* **93**:163–6.

Chalmers, I, Enkin, M and Keirse, M J N C (1989). *Effective Care in Pregnancy and Childbirth*. Oxford: Oxford University Press.

Cook, T D and Campbell, D T (1979). *Quasi-experimentation: design and analysis issues for field settings*. Boston, Massachusetts: Houghton Mifflin.

Cousins, J H, Rubovits, D S, Dunn, J K, Reeves, R S, Ramirez, A G and Foreyt, J P (1992). Family versus individually oriented intervention for weight loss in Mexican American women. *Public Health Reports* **107**:549–55.

Cox, R H, Parker, G G, Watson, A C, Robinson, S H, Simonson, C J, Elledge, J C, Diggs, S and Smith, M (1995). Dietary cancer risk of low-income women and change with intervention. *American Dietetic Association Journal* **95**:1031–4.

Cucherat, M and Boissel, J P (1993). Meta-analysis of results of clinical trials on prevention of coronary heart disease by lipid-lowering interventions. *Clinical Trials and Meta-Analysis* **28**:109–29.

Czeizel, A E (1993). Prevention of congenital abnormalities by peri-conceptional multivitamin supplementation. *British Medical Journal* **306**:1645–8.

Czeizel, A E and Dudas, I (1992). Prevention of the first occurrence of neural-tube defects by periconceptional vitamin supplementation. *New England Journal of Medicine* **327**:1832–5.

Devine, C M and Olson, C M (1992). Women's perceptions about the way social roles promote or constrain personal nutrition care. *Women & Health* **19**:79–95.

Devine, C M and Sandstrom, B (1996). Relationship of social roles and nutrition beliefs to fat avoidance practices: investigation of a US model among Danish women. *American Dietetic Association Journal* **96**:580–4.

Donner, A, Birkett, N and Buck, C (1981). Randomisation by cluster: sample size requirements and analysis. *American Journal of Epidemiology* **114**:906–94.

Donner, A and Donald, A (1987). Analysis of data arising from a stratified design with the cluster as unit of randomisation. *Statistics in Medicine* **6**:43–52.

Dow Allen, C and Ries, C P (1985). Smoking, alcohol, and dietary practices during pregnancy: comparison before and after prenatal education. *American Dietetic Association Journal* **85**:605–6.

Doyle, W (1996). Women and health: nutritional and psychological factors. In: Buttriss, J and Hyman, K (eds). *Focus on women*. London: National Dairy Council.

Doyle, W, Wynn, A H A, Crawford, M A and Wynn, S W (1992). Nutritional counselling and supplementation in the second and third trimester of pregnancy: a study in a London population. *Journal of Nutritional Medicine* **3**:249–56.

Dubois, S, Dougherty, C, Duquette, M P, Hanley, J A and Mountquin, J M (1991). Twin pregnancy: the impact of the Higgins Nutrition Intervention Program on maternal and neonatal outcomes. *American Journal of Clinical Nutrition* **53**:1397–1403.

Edwards, C R W, Benedicktsson, R, Lindsay, R S and Seckl, J R (1993). Dysfunction of placental glucocorticoid barrier: link between fetal environment and adult hypertension. *Lancet* **341**:355–7.

Edwards, P, Acock, A C and Johnson, R L (1985). Nutrition behaviour change: outcomes of an educational approach. *Evaluation Review* **9**:441–59.

Ernst, N D, Wu, M, Frommer, P, Katz, E, Matthews, O, Moskowitz, J, Pinsky, J L, Pohl, S, Schreiber, G B and Sondik, E (1986). Nutrition education at the point of purchase. *Preventive Medicine* **15**:60–73.

Fine, G A, Conning, D M, Firmin, C, de Looy, A E, Losowsky, M S, Richards, I D G and Webster, J (1994). Nutrition education of young women. *British Journal of Nutrition* **71**:789–98.

Flynn, M A T (1996). Are national dietary guidelines for healthy eating suitable for women? In: Buttriss, J and Hyman, K (eds). *Focus on Women*. London: National Dairy Council.

Fraser, A M, Brockert, J E and Ward, R H (1995). Association of young maternal age with adverse reproductive outcomes. *New England Journal of Medicine* **332**:1113–17.

Fugate Woods, N (1991). The research agenda model as a framework for research about women and nutrition. *American Journal of Health Promotion* **5**:222–5.

Galletly, C, Clark, A, Tomlinson, L and Blaney, F (1996). Improved pregnancy rates for obese, infertile women following a group treatment program: an open pilot study. *General Hospital Psychiatry* **18**:192–5.

Godfrey, K M, Redman, C W G, Barker, D J P and Osmond, C (1995). The effect of maternal anaemia and iron deficiency on the ratio of fetal weight to placental weight. *Reproduction, Fertility and Development* **7**:333–44.

Goode, J, Beardsworth, A, Keil, T, Sherrat, E and Haslam, C (1994). Changing the nation's diet: a study of responses to current nutritional messages. *Health Education Journal* **55**:285–99.

Health Education Authority Coronary Prevention Group (1993). *Nutrition interventions in primary health care: a literature review*. London: HEA.

Heins, H C, Nance, N W, McCarthy, B J and Efird, C M (1990). A randomized trial of nurse-midwifery pre-natal care to reduce low birth weight. *Obstetrics and Gynecology* **75**:341–5.

Herman, A A, Berendes, H W, Yu, K F, Cooper, C, Overpeck, M D, Rhoads, G, Maxwell, J P, Kinney, B A, Koslowe, P A and Coates, D L (1996). Evaluation of the effectiveness of a community-based enriched model prenatal intervention project in the District of Columbia. *Health Services Research* **31**:609–21.

Higgins, A (1976). Nutritional status and the outcome of pregnancy. *Journal of the Canadian Dietetic Association* **36**:17–35.

Johnson, Z, Howell, F and Molloy, B (1993). Community mothers' programme: randomised controlled trial of non-professional intervention in parenting. *British Medical Journal* **306**:1449–52.

Kafatos, A G, Tsitoura, S, Pantelakis, S N and Doxiadis, S A (1991). Maternal and infant health education in a rural Greek community. *Hygie* **10**:32–7.

Kafatos, A G, Vlachonikolis, I G and Codrington, C A (1989). Nutrition during pregnancy: the effects of an educational intervention program in Greece. *American Journal of Clinical Nutrition* **50**:970–9.

Kafatos, A G, Vlachonikolis, I G, Codrington, C A and Belsey, M (1993). Nutrition during pregnancy: the effects of an educational intervention program in Greece. *American Journal of Clinical Nutrition* **50**:970–9.

Keim, N L, Canty, D J, Barbieri, T F and Wu, M M (1996). Effect of exercise and dietary restraint on energy intake of reduced-obese women. *Appetite* **26**:55–70.

Kennett, D J and Ackerman, M (1995). Importance of learned resourcefulness to weight loss and early success during maintenance: preliminary evidence. *Patient Education and Counseling* **25**:197–203.

Kramer, M S (1993). Effects of energy and protein intakes on pregnancy outcome: an overview of the research evidence from controlled clinical trials. *American Journal of Clinical Nutrition* **58**:627–35.

Kumanyika, S K and Charleston, J B (1992). Lose weight and win: a church based weight loss program for blood pressure control among black women. *Patient Education and Counseling* **19**:19–32.

Langer, A, Victora, C, Victora, M, Barros, F, Farnot, U, Belizán, J and Villar, J (1993). The Latin American trial of psychosocial support during pregnancy: a social intervention evaluated through an experimental design. *Social Science and Medicine* **36**:495–507.

Larsson, I and Lissner, L (1996). The Green Keyhole nutritional campaign in Sweden: Do women with more knowledge have better dietary practices? *European Journal of Clinical Nutrition* **50**:323–8.

Lia-Hoagberg, B, Rode, P and Skovholt, C J (1990). Barriers and motivators to prenatal care among low-income women. *Social Science and Medicine* **30**:487–95.

Liedekerken, P C, Jonkers, R, de Haes, W F M, Kok, J G and Saan, J M (1990). *Effectiveness of health education: review and analysis*. Assen, The Netherlands: Van Gorcum Uitgeverij.

Lissner, L, Bengtsson, C, Bjorkelund, C and Wedel, H (1996). Physical activity levels and changes in relation to longevity: a prospective study of Swedish women. *American Journal of Epidemiology* **143**:54–62.

Loris, P, Dewey, K G and Poirier-Brode, K (1985). Weight gain and dietary intake of pregnant teenagers. *American Dietetic Association Journal* **85**:1296–1305.

McCargar, L, Taunton, J, Birmingham, C L, Pare, S and Simmons, D (1993). Metabolic and anthropometric changes in female weight cyclers and controls over a 1-year period. *American Dietetic Association Journal* **93**:1025–30.

McEnery, G and Rao, K P S (1986). The effectiveness of antenatal education of Pakistani and Indian women living in this country. *Child: Care, Health and Development* **12**:385–99.

Medical Research Council Vitamin Study Research Group, Wald, N (1991). Prevention of neural tube defects: results of the Medical Research Council Vitamin Study. *Lancet* **338**:131–7.

Megel, M E, Wade, F, Hawkins, P and Norton, J (1994). Health promotion, self-esteem, and weight among female college freshmen. *Health Values* **18**:10–19.

A meta-analysis and synthesis of nutrition education research(1985). *Journal of Nutrition Education* **17**:S11–S19.

Metcoff, J, Costiloe, P, Crosby, W M, Dutta, S, Sandstead, H H, Milne, D, Bodwell, C E and Majors, S H (1985). Effect of food supplementation (WIC) during pregnancy on birth weight. *American Journal of Clinical Nutrition* **41**:933–47.

Metson, D, Kremer, G, Tobin, M, Kassianos, G, Norman, D, Moriarty, J, Jones, M, Bloomfield, C and Cruse, J (1996). Promoting folic acid intake during pregnancy. *Audit in General Practice* **4**:13–15.

Monsen, E and Cheney, C (1988). Research methods in nutrition and dietetics: design, data analysis, and presentation. *American Dietetic Association Journal* **88**:1047–65.

NHS Centre for Reviews and Dissemination (1996). *Undertaking systematic reviews of research on effectiveness: CRD guidelines for those carrying out or commissioning reviews.* CRD report 4. York: NHS CRD.

National Advisory Committee on Nutrition Education (NACNE) (1983). *Proposals for nutritional guidelines for health education in Britain.* London: Health Education Council.

National Cholesterol Education Program (NCEP) (1993). Expert panel on detection evaluation and treatment of high blood cholesterol in adults. *Journal of the American Medical Association* **269**:3015–29.

National Institute of Health. Consensus development panel on optimal calcium intake (1994). *Journal of the American Medical Association* **272**:1942–7

Nunn, R G, Newton, K S and Faucher, P (1992). 2.5 years follow up of weight and body mass index values in the Weight Control for Life! Program: a descriptive analysis. *Addictive Behaviors* **17**:579–85.

Olsen, S F, Sorensen, J D, Secher, N J, Hedegaard, M, Henriksen, T B, Hansen, H S and Grant, A (1992). Randomized controlled trial of effect of fish-oil supplementation on pregnancy duration. *Lancet* **339**:1003–7.

Orstead, C, Arrington, D, Kamath, S K, Olson, R and Kohrs, M B (1985). Efficacy of prenatal nutrition counseling: weight gain, infant birth weight, and cost-effectiveness. *American Dietetic Association Journal* **85**:40–5.

Perkin, J (1983). Evaluating a nutrition education program for pregnant teenagers: cognitive vs behavioral outcomes. *Journal of School Health* **53**:420–2.

Portsmouth, K, Henderson, K, Graham, N, Price, R, Cole, J and Allen, J (1994). Dietary calcium intake in 18 year old women: comparison with recommended daily intake and dietary energy intake. *Journal of Advanced Nursing* **20**:1073–8.

Powell, J J, Tucker, L, Fisher, A G and Wilcox, K (1994). The effects of different percentages of dietary fat intake, exercise, and calorie restriction on body composition and body weight in obese females. *American Journal of Health Promotion* **8**: 442–8.

Quinn, T J and Jenkins, M (1991). Nutritional profiles of selected college females in a 15-week exercise and weight control class. *Health Values* **15**:34–41.

Reinli, K, Will, K, Thompson, Reid, P, Liburd, P and Anderson, L A (1996). Predicting barriers to healthy eating and physical activity among black women. *Journal of Women's Health* **5**:51–9.

Research Information Systems (1995). *Reference Manager, Professional Edition 7.01.* Carlsbad, California: Research Information Systems.

Rush, D (1986). Nutrition in the preparation for pregnancy. In: Chamberlain, G and Lumley, J (eds). *Pre-pregnancy care: a manual for practice.* London: John Wiley.

Rush, D, Alvir, J M, Kenny, D A, Johnson, S S and Horvitz, D G (1988a). The National WIC Evaluation: evaluation of the Special Supplemental Food Program for Women, Infants, and Children, III. Historical study of pregnancy outcomes. *American Journal of Clinical Nutrition* **48**(2 suppl):412–28.

Rush, D, Horvitz, D G, Seaver, W B, Alvir, J M, Garbowski, G C, Leighton, J, Sloan, N L, Johnson, S S, Kulka, R A and Shanklin, D S (1988b). The National WIC Evaluation: evaluation of the Special Supplemental Food Program for Women, Infants, and Children, I. Background and introduction. *American Journal of Clinical Nutrition* **48**(2 suppl): 389–93.

Rush, D, Horvitz, D G, Seaver, W B, Leighton, J, Sloan, N L, Johnson, S S, Kulka, R A, Devore, J W, Holt, M, Lynch, J T *et al.* (1988c). The National WIC Evaluation: evaluation of the Special Supplemental Food Program for Women, Infants, and Children, IV. Study methodology and sample characteristics in the longitudinal study of pregnant women, the study of children, and the food expenditures study. *American Journal of Clinical Nutrition* **48**(2 suppl):429–38.

Rush, D, Leighton, J, Sloan, N L, Alvir, J M and Garbowski, G C (1988d). The National WIC Evaluation: evaluation of the Special Supplemental Food Program for Women, Infants, and Children, II. Review of past studies of WIC. *American Journal of Clinical Nutrition* **48**(2 suppl):394–411.

Rush, D, Sloan, N L, Leighton, J, Alvir, J M, Horvitz, D G, Seaver, W B, Garbowski, G C, Johnson, S S, Kulka, R A and Holt, M (1988e). The National WIC Evaluation: evaluation of the Special Supplemental Food Program for Women, Infants, and Children, V. Longitudinal study of pregnant women. *American Journal of Clinical Nutrition* **48**(2 suppl):439–83.

Sackett, D L, Haynes, R B and Tugwell, P (1985). *Clinical epidemiology: a basic science for clinicians.* New York: Little, Brown.

Schofield, E C, Wheeler, E F and Stewart, J D (1988). Is the message getting through? Nutritional knowledge of pregnant women in Edinburgh and London. *European Journal of Clinical Nutrition* **42**:161–7.

Schramm, W F (1985). WIC prenatal participation and its relationship to newborn Medicaid costs in Missouri: a cost/benefit analysis. *American Journal of Public Health* **75**:851–7.

Schramm, W F (1986). Prenatal participation in WIC related to Medicaid costs for Missouri newborns: 1982 update. *Public Health Reports* **101**:607–15.

Shah, M, Baxter, J E, McGovern, P G and Garg, A (1996). Nutrient and food intake in obese women on a low-fat or low-calorie diet. *American Journal of Health Promotion* **10**:179–82.

Simkin-Silverman, L, Wing, R and Hansen, D H (1995). Prevention of cardiovascular risk factor elevations in healthy premenopausal women. *Preventive Medicine* **24**:509–17.

Skeoch, H, Skeoch C, Rosenberg K, Turner T and McIlwaine, G (1987). Very low birthweight survivors: illness and readmission to hospital in the first 15 months of life. *British Medical Journal* **295**:579–80.

Smith, P J, Moffatt, E K, Gelskey, S C *et al.* (1997). Are community health interventions evaluated appropriately? A review of six journals. *Journal of Clinical Epidemiology* **50**:137–46.

Stockbauer, J W (1986). Evaluation of the Missouri WIC program: prenatal components. *American Dietetic Association Journal* **86**:61–7.

Stockbauer, J W (1987). WIC prenatal participation and its relation to pregnancy outcomes in Missouri: a second look. *American Journal of Public Health* **77**:813–18.

Sutherland, H J, Carlin, K, Harper, W and Martin, L J (1993). A study of diet and breast cancer prevention in Canada: why healthy women participate in controlled trials. *Cancer Causes and Control* **4**:521–8.

Sweeney, C, Smith, H, Foster, J C, Place, J C, Specht, J, Kochenour, N K and Prater, B M (1985). Effects of a nutrition intervention program during pregnancy: maternal data, Phases 1 and 2. *Journal of Nurse Midwifery* **30**:149–58.

Taren, D L and Graven, S N (1991). The association of prenatal nutrition and educational services with low birth weight rates in a Florida program. *Public Health Reports* **106**:426–36.

Trouba, P H, Okereke, N and Splett, P L (1991). Summary document of nutrition intervention in prenatal care. *American Dietetic Association Journal* suppl: S21–6.

Tucker, L A, Harris, K and Martin, J R (1996). Participation in a strength training program leads to improved dietary intake in adult women. *American Dietetic Association Journal* **96**:388–90.

Villar, J, Farnot, U, Barros, F, Victora, C, Langer, A and Belizán, J M (1992). A randomized trial of psychosocial support during high risk pregnancies. *New England Journal of Medicine* **327**:1266–71.

Wallace, J M, Aitken, R P and Cheyne, M A (1994). Effect of post-ovulation nutritional status in ewes on early conceptus survival and growth in vivo and luteotrophic protein secretion in vitro. *Reproduction, Fertility and Development* **6**:253–9.

Whitehead, M (1991). *Avoiding the pitfalls: notes on the planning and implementation of health education strategies and the special role of the HEA*. London: Health Education Authority.

Whiting-O'Keefe, Q E, Henke, C and Simborg, D W (1984). Choosing the correct unit of analysis in medical care experiments. *Medical Care* **22**:1101–14.

World Health Organization (1995). Maternal anthropometry and pregnancy outcomes: a WHO collaborative project. *Bulletin* **73**:supplement.